Acclaim for *Hope Amid the Pain*

Beautifully written, *Hope Amid the Pain* tugs at the heart with both practical and spiritual instruction. Anyone who is or has suffered with crippling and debilitating pain or illness will find encouragement and support in this devotional. Spirit lifting, wise, and filled with inspiration, this devotional is sure to strengthen hearts for wherever the Lord is leading.

Debbie Macomber | #1 NYT bestselling author

With poignant and practical words, Leslie is able to reach into someone's heart and give it a squeeze while at the same time holding their hand and giving them the strength and wisdom they need to get through their day. *Hope Amid The Pain* is the devotional book women have been waiting for. With powerful messages about hope, you can't help but get chills as you read her encouraging words.

Rachel Van Dyken | #1 NYT bestselling author

McKee writes with compassion and understanding. Words of grace and compassion for those struggling with chronic pain.

Vannetta Chapman | *USA Today* bestselling author

As a mental health therapist I often look for resources for clients who struggle with chronic mental and physical illnesses. Leslie L. McKee speaks from personal experience as a woman who suffers from chronic illness. She has combined her personal experience, her deep faith in Christ, and her writing skills to provide a devotional which will truly minister to women who are fellow travelers on the chronic illness journey. Her format provides encouragement with practical application based on Scripture. I can't wait to be able to offer such a devotional to my clients.

Patricia J Edwards | LCSW, The Antioch Group

With compassion and hope, Leslie L. McKee offers a glimpse into her own journey through chronic illness and pain that many readers will relate to. Each day's reading leads with edifying scripture and finishes with an opportunity for the reader to respond. With a unique focus on walking bravely through chronic illness and pain, this book would make a great gift for a friend or family member. Since there is an increasing number in today's society struggling with the stigma and loneliness of chronic illness and pain, *HOPE Amid the Pain* could become a powerful tool and companion to many.

Elizabeth Byler Younts | author of Carol Award Winning *The Solace of Water*

Sometimes we just need a friend to put their arms around us and whisper "I've been there, too." Through the pages of *Hope Amid the Pain*, Leslie L. McKee is that friend—coming alongside fellow chronic illness warriors with compassion and vulnerability. Leslie's honesty in sharing her own journey through chronic illness and the biblical reflections filling every page are gifts to the reader. Rich with truth, encouragement, and hope, these devotions are a balm to hearts weary from suffering.

Amanda Barratt | author of *The White Rose Resists* and *My Dearest Dietrich*

With an understanding heart born of years of her own experience fighting chronic pain, Leslie L. McKee encourages readers with sixty beautiful, biblical devotions that will inspire, encourage, and help those of us suffering with illness to glimpse an eternal perspective and hope not of this world. Saturated in truth, *Hope Amid the Pain* helps readers silence the lies of fear and doubt by practicing gratitude and reminding themselves of their true identity in Christ. I highly recommend this devotional for anyone who has felt the frustration of chronic pain.

Heidi Chiavaroli | award-winning author of *Freedom's Ring* and *The Tea Chest*

Leslie L. McKee has penned a valuable resource for those who suffer with chronic illnesses. I am one of those people and wished I'd had this book when I was first diagnosed. The daily suggestions on how to rely on God in the midst of such suffering and the resource guide in the back are priceless. I highly recommend *Hope Amid the Pain*.

Susan Sleeman | bestselling author of the *Truth Seekers* and *Homeland Heroes* series

Hope Amid the Pain is an inspiring, relevant devotional that is filled with comfort and encouragement. A must-have for anyone struggling with chronic illness.

Kathleen Fuller | bestselling author of the *Amish of Birch Creek* series

Hope Amid the Pain should be prescribed to anyone suffering with a health condition. It is the kind of book that makes you want to holler out "AMEN!" after each day's devotion. Unexpected health concerns sweep the rug right out from under the patient and their families. They need compassion and understanding, and Leslie L. McKee provides that. She also shares her own experiences, adding validity to the daily encouragement. *Hope Amid the Pain* reminds the reader they are not alone, and most of all, there is hope that God will use the time of suffering for His glory.

Sharee Stover | author with Love Inspired Suspense

You are loved. You are not alone. You are worthy. For those suffering with chronic pain or illness, there is no more merciful balm. McKee's 60-day devotional offers Scripture that encourages reflection, practical advice, resources, and helpful hacks for managing disappointment, pain, and uncertainty. Poignant, sometimes humorous personal insights from the author's twenty-five years as a chronic pain warrior add to the reader's sense of empathy and support. A valuable resource toward living a hope-filled life.

Candace Calvert | award-winning author of hopeful medical fiction

Leslie L. McKee's *Hope Amid the Pain: Hanging On to Positive Expectations When Battling Chronic Pain and Illness, A 60-Day Devotional Journal* is an inspiring, spiritual journey of encouragement. Leslie L. McKee's personal stories, along with her advice, tips, and hacks are just what readers need in order to feel the power of grace and hope and, above all, an unfailing faith in God's Word and His promises.

Amy Clipston | bestselling author of *The Farm Stand*

LESLIE L. MCKEE

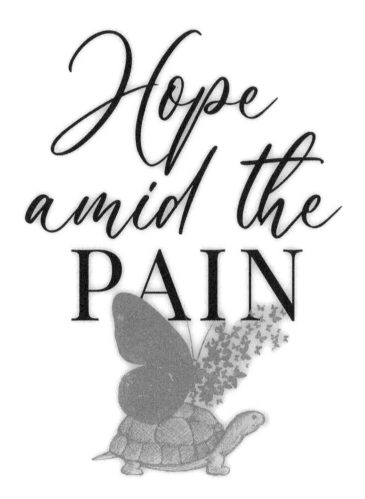

Hope amid the PAIN

HANGING ON TO POSITIVE EXPECTATIONS

WHEN BATTLING CHRONIC PAIN AND ILLNESS

A 60-DAY DEVOTIONAL JOURNAL

Ambassador International
GREENVILLE, SOUTH CAROLINA & BELFAST, NORTHERN IRELAND

www.ambassador-international.com

Hope Amid the Pain

Hanging On to Positive Expectations When Battling Chronic Pain and Illness (a 60-Day Devotional Journal)

Hardcover ISBN: 978-1-64960-215-2
Paperback ISBN: 978-1-64960-132-2
eISBN: 978-1-64960-182-7

Cover Design by Hannah Linder Designs
Interior Design by Dentelle Design
Edited by Katie Cruice Smith

Holy Bible, New Living Translation, copyright © 1996, 2004, 2015 by Tyndale House Foundation. Used by permission of Tyndale House Publishers, Inc., Carol Stream, Illinois 60188. All rights reserved.

AMBASSADOR INTERNATIONAL
Emerald House
411 University Ridge, Suite B14
Greenville, SC 29601, USA
www.ambassador-international.com

AMBASSADOR BOOKS
The Mount
2 Woodstock Link
Belfast, BT6 8DD, Northern Ireland, UK
www.ambassadormedia.co.uk

The colophon is a trademark of Ambassador, a Christian publishing company.

To Oram:

Thank you for your love and encouragement and for always being one of my biggest supporters. I'm so blessed by the many years we've had together, and I'm honored to share my writing with you. I love you so very much.

Table of Contents

INTRODUCTION

And we know that God causes everything to work together for the good of those who love God and are called according to his purpose for them.

—Romans 8:28

God promises to use *all things* for His good. For those living with chronic pain and illness, it could be hard to believe that's true. But He sees the big picture. He offers hope for those who feel hopeless, comfort in times of trouble, courage to squash fears, and strength to take that next step.

Dear friend, I don't know what you're going through, and I don't presume to know how you feel. But I do know what it's like to live with chronic pain and illness. I know what it's like to question God and wonder why others are healed while I'm still in pain. Yet I also know where to turn when I feel like I can't continue and am ready to give up. I know where to find strength to take that next step, and I know where to find hope for the future. All of it can be found in one place—in one person—Jesus, the One *Who is Hope*!

With *HOPE Amid the Pain*, I share some Scripture verses, quotes, and perspectives that have helped me over the twenty-five-plus years I've dealt with chronic pain and illness. I pray that you can find hope and comfort in these pages when the waves of life threaten to overwhelm you. (To learn more about me and my battle, see "My Story" at the back of the book.)

Life is full of choices. You can choose to be unhappy with your situation, or you can grab on to hope and live the best life possible. It's impossible to change the past, and you have little influence over the reactions of others. When you are living with chronic pain and illness, your life may often seem out of control. There will be some things you can do nothing about, no matter how hard you try. However, you can always control your attitude and perspective.

Chronic pain is a thief. It steals your time and productivity. You may lose some of your abilities as well as your sense of self. But it doesn't steal your true identity. You are *not* your pain or your illness. You have a disorder. It may even be a neurobiological one, which means it's caused by genetic or metabolic factors. Having physical limitations doesn't make you a less-valuable person. You still have a purpose. Your illness does *not* define you, even though it may, on occasion, confine you. It doesn't determine your worth or value. God does. You are enough just as you are.

This book is not a cure. It's a reminder that you're not alone. As a Christ-follower, these devotions can serve as a reminder that you can hold on to hope because you know Jesus. Chronic pain and illness are always changing. Blessedly, the Lord is constant.

Though it may be hard to believe in the moment, God *does* have a plan. He can use everything—even that pain you see no purpose for, the pain you think holds you back. Let me tell you a secret—it doesn't! *You are an overcomer.* A survivor. A child of the Most High. You have strength others—perhaps even yourself—may not see, but God does. He has given you a message to share with others that no one else can tell.

Somewhere along the line, the enemy's lies may have replaced God's truths. It's possible that you have settled for just getting by rather than living your life. My hope with this devotional is to remind you that you are valuable, you are worthy, and you are loved. I pray the devotions will draw you closer to God's words so that you can find comfort and strength. I hope the questions included with each devotion provide you with an opportunity to reflect and listen to what God may want to say to you. This book is a reminder that it's okay to embrace hope and dream again. I want you to look in the mirror and see your situation in a different light. I pray you can view yourself the way

God sees you: as His daughter and His beloved. You may have a chronic illness or chronic pain, but you are not ruined beyond repair. There is beauty in the brokenness. Will this change in your mindset happen overnight? Probably not. But I pray that by the time you finish this book (whether it's the seventh time or even the seventieth time), you will understand a few things:

- You are *not* defined by your pain, illness, or disability.
- Your *hope* does not depend on your physical or mental health.
- You are *perfectly imperfect.*
- You are *unique and special.*
- You are *never alone.*
- You *can do everything* with Christ.
- You *are loved* by the Lord.

DAY 1

Unfinished

And I am certain that God, who began the good work within you,
will continue his work until it is finally finished on the day when Christ Jesus returns.

—Philippians 1:6

Growing up, did you ever think about the future and where you would be at this stage of your life? I know I did. I had great plans—so many things I wanted to be and do. However, everything didn't turn out as I envisioned. Oh sure, some things did, and some even turned out better than I expected. I certainly never thought I'd be dealing with chronic pain and chronic illness, struggling some days to do the most basic tasks. Saying no to activities I'd love to do because my body is telling me I can't. Watching family and friends have fun while I sit on the sidelines.

In today's verse, Paul was speaking to the people of Philippi. He viewed them through eyes of faith. He was able to encourage them because he saw them as they would be when God was finished with them, not as they currently were.

It's easy to focus on how things didn't go as planned and to get depressed. That's a natural response to grief and loss, particularly in response to chronic pain and illness. However, Philippians 1:6 is a wonderful reminder that while you may not be where you want to be or thought you'd be, God's not finished with you yet. You can be confident that God has begun a good work in you, and He will perform it until the day Jesus returns. Life may not be as you envisioned, but you can be certain that God has a plan for you. Be thankful for what you *can* do and *have* done instead of focusing on what you can't do or haven't done. Abide in the Lord daily. Like the Philippians, you are a work in progress—God's beautiful creation. Nothing, not even chronic pain and illness, can change that.

Lord, I know Your plan for me is perfect, and I will find rest in that knowledge. Amen.

Reflection

What have you done that you can be thankful for today?

_____

_____

_____

_____

_____

_____

_____

_____

_____

_____

_____

_____

DAY 2

The Gift of Peace

I am leaving you with a gift—peace of mind and heart. And the peace I give is a gift the world cannot give. So don't be troubled or afraid.

—John 14:27

Peace. It seems like such an elusive concept. Some days, I can barely sit still. There always seems to be something I should be working on or doing. And my mind? That's another thing altogether. It fires on all cylinders most of the time. My husband tells me that "relax" isn't part of my vocabulary. But that doesn't stop me from chasing after peace, though I often find it difficult to grab. How about you?

In today's verse, we are promised a peace unlike anything we can receive elsewhere. Jesus suffered, but He still offered peace. That peace is our inheritance. It's what Jesus left us. Circumstances cannot take it away. That's what is meant by the phrase, "And the peace I give is a gift the world cannot give." It's a peace that passes *all* understanding. It's hard for me to even wrap my mind around that concept. As I sit here with tense muscles and racing thoughts, I think about the image of peace—and it sounds wonderful. It's exactly what I need. But can I allow myself to accept it? Can you?

Doing so would mean letting go and allowing God to have control. That's hard for many, myself included. But the facets of chronic pain and illness are beyond human control. That phrase means letting go and giving God control of the thoughts that say, *You should be doing this* or *If you would only do that.* It is possible to walk in God's peace, but it's a choice that must be made each and every day. His peace is possible in any situation, even the painful ones. Don't let the enemy win control of your mind. Accept God's gift of peace today.

Lord, when my body and mind tell me otherwise, let me cling to the peace You are offering me at this moment. Amen.

Reflection

What steps can you take today toward accepting God's gift of peace?

_____

_____

_____

_____

_____

_____

_____

_____

_____

_____

_____

_____

_____

_____

DAY 3

Priceless

The Lord will hold you in his hand for all to see—
a splendid crown in the hand of God.

—Isaiah 62:3

Have you ever seen the discount rack at a store? It often contains out-of-fashion items or clothing with slight flaws. I once bought a shirt with thread a slightly different color on the hem. It really wasn't noticeable unless you were examining the item closely. However, that tiny flaw allowed me to purchase the item at a significantly reduced price because it was deemed "damaged" by the store.

Have you ever felt damaged? I know I have, especially on days when I'm having a flare-up. "I'm not as thin as she is." "I'm not as pretty as my friend." "I can't do what she can do." "My limitations make me a burden to my loved ones." Do similar thoughts ever pop into your head? It's easy to fall into the comparison game, but it leads only to insecurity and stress. That, in turn, adds to increased pain. It's truly a vicious cycle, yet it's one many people go through daily.

Can I tell you something? It's a reminder I tell myself on a regular basis. Those thoughts you tell yourself? They aren't how God sees you, and that's not how He wants you to see yourself either. As today's verse states, you are a "splendid crown" in God's hand—extremely valuable. Crowns are made out of gemstones, which are formed by a great amount of pressure. People are formed in a similar way. The Lord uses your challenges, including your pain, to shape you. Your beauty shines through the One Who holds you. You are a reflection of Him. Nothing you do or don't do will change His opinion of you. Remember that as you look in your mirror today.

Lord, help me to see the potential and beauty that You see in me. Amen.

Reflection

What is God showing you in the mirror today?

_____

_____

_____

_____

_____

_____

_____

_____

_____

_____

_____

_____

_____

DAY 4

Labor Pains

Yet what we suffer now is nothing compared to the glory he will reveal to us later.

—Romans 8:18

I can't imagine meeting someone who would admit that they enjoy pain and suffering. However, most people would agree that pain is something we all go through on occasion. Many times, something good comes from that experience—though it's not always recognized in the moment.

When we experience pain, we try to alleviate it or make sense of it. The same is often true when we see others in pain. Take a woman experiencing labor pains. If you've ever witnessed this, there is no doubt giving birth is a painful experience. In the moment, the soon-to-be mom would attest to that. However, ask her days, or even years, later—when she's holding her beautiful child—and she's likely to view that once-painful moment (delivery) in a different light because so much joy came out of that period of pain.

The New Testament often speaks of the incomparable glory that lies ahead for us. Today's verse is a reminder from Paul that pain and suffering shouldn't be our focus. Paul was speaking from experience, as he suffered immensely. Despite being stoned, imprisoned, shipwrecked, and starved, he knew that couldn't compare to the joy ahead. He never gave up hope in that fact. Pain and suffering last for a moment—though they may seem everlasting at the time—but "joy comes with the morning" (Psalm 30:5). God was there in the midst of your last trial, and He brought you through it. He will not abandon you. He'll bring you through this one and the next one as well. In His time, God will shed light on the purpose behind your pain. Look to Him now to see you through it.

Lord, I may not understand why I'm experiencing this situation, but I know
You are here with me, carrying me through to the joy on the other side. Amen.

Reflection

When did God bring you through a trial?

_____

_____

_____

_____

_____

_____

_____

_____

_____

_____

_____

_____

_____

DAY 5

Open Arms

Let all that I am wait quietly before God, for my hope is in him.

—Psalm 62:5

I have fond memories of staying at my grandparents' house as a child. I also remember being scared of thunderstorms. I was okay with the rumbles, but the lightning was a different story. Crawling into bed beside my gram and resting in her arms helped. She would tell me I had nothing to fear. The sounds I heard were God bowling. (By the way, He got lots of strikes!) It may seem silly now, but as a child, that analogy helped ease my fears. I was no longer afraid because I trusted that Gram would keep me safe and comfort me. Our Father God is the same way.

Today's verse tells us to "wait quietly before God." That's not always easy during flare-ups. It's hard to concentrate on anything else when pain screams for attention. You may even feel that everything is spiraling out of control. People are depending on you, yet you can barely focus on taking your next breath. In those moments, you can do like King David did and find your hope in the Lord. This verse was a reminder to David to look to and trust God, and it can be a reminder to you, too.

Chronic pain can sometimes make a person feel scared, anxious, alone, or even helpless. It may feel like it's beyond your human control, and on occasion, it is. However, it's never too much for God. Hope and security can always be found in Him. God wants us to go to Him for refuge, comfort, and peace. So, the next time you feel that you can't cope, that you're scared, or that life is overwhelming, allow yourself to run to Him and hunker down in God's open, loving arms. He's there reaching out to you. Find your rest and hope in Him.

Lord, today I place my hope in You as I am wrapped in Your arms. Amen.

Reflection

What's something that makes you feel secure?

_____

_____

_____

_____

_____

_____

_____

_____

_____

_____

_____

_____

_____

DAY 6

Through God's Eyes

See how very much our Father loves us, for he calls us his children, and that is what we are!

—1 John 3:1

Tonight's the concert. We've been waiting months for this. I sure hope I don't ruin it. I just want one pain-free evening. Those and other similar thoughts went through my head as I woke up with a fibromyalgia flare-up and migraine. It's challenging for me to be around crowds on a good day, as I never know when or if the fragrances, lighting, or sounds will be a trigger. I'm even more concerned when I wake up with my nerves and pain already firing.

Those who suffer from chronic pain and illness are familiar with sitting on the sidelines, watching others participate in the dance party, game of catch, movie, or other activities their friends and family members are doing. Society often has little room for people with "blemishes." They may view us as "less than," which skews our self-identity, making us wonder who we are and what our purpose is. Thankfully, God's view is vastly different than society's.

Being a child of God is a powerful source of strength and hope. There is a sense of peace in the knowledge that we're not alone in our pain. We are accepted and loved just as we are—and that includes our illness and pain. Our Father's love is unconditional. We don't need to do anything to make Him love us more. There is security in that knowledge. No matter what physical issue we have, God sees us as valuable and precious. We were purchased with

29

the blood of His Son. We are His child, and *nothing*—not even chronic pain or illness—can ever change that.

> *Lord, when pain or society distorts my self-image, remind me that I'm*
> *Your beloved daughter and help me see myself as You see me. Amen.*

Reflection

What distorted vision of yourself can you cast aside today, knowing that you're valuable to God?

_____

_____

_____

_____

_____

_____

_____

_____

_____

_____

_____

_____

_____

_____

DAY 7

Have Patience

Rejoice in our confident hope. Be patient in trouble, and keep on praying.

—Romans 12:12

Paul's directives in this verse caught my eye one day during my morning devotional time. I could barely turn my neck or take a deep breath without pain. No doubt about it. I was in the midst of a flare-up. I looked back at today's verse. Paul was telling me to be joyful and patient. Seriously? I almost laughed at how impossible that sounded. Then I remembered how Paul experienced trials I couldn't begin to imagine. Even then, he was still able to rejoice. How was that possible?

Upon further reflection, I realized three things about this verse. First, Paul wasn't asking me to be happy about my pain. He was telling me to be joyful in my hope—the hope found only in Jesus. For Christ-followers, the future is secure, as evidenced by His resurrection.

Next, Paul says to "be patient in trouble." To be patient means to withstand pains or trials calmly and without complaint. I'll admit that patience isn't one of my strong points, and it may not be one of yours either. However, Paul shares this reminder: God isn't finished with me—or you—yet. As it states in James 1:2-4, struggles, suffering, and other tests develop perseverance and faith.

Finally, Paul asks us to pray. Prayer releases God's power in our lives. Not only are we asked to pray, but we're also asked to "keep on praying." We should be in constant conversation with God on a regular daily basis. We are called to His purpose, so we can pray and cry out to Him in confidence. By faith, we can trust that God will hear us, and He will answer—in His time and in accordance to His will (Mark 11:24). Stress and anxiety increase pain, frustration, and a host of other negatives. None of them will change the timetable of God's plans. So, place your hope in God and live each day to the fullest, giving what you are able to give each day.

Lord, today I choose to live my life to the fullest, with my hope placed firmly in You. Amen.

Reflection

In what area do you need a bit of patience today?

_____

_____

_____

_____

_____

_____

_____

_____

_____

_____

_____

_____

_____

_____

DAY 8

Strong Tower

From the ends of the earth, I cry to you for help when my heart is overwhelmed. Lead me to the towering rock of safety, for you are my safe refuge, a fortress where my enemies cannot reach me.

—Psalm 61:2-3

Life can feel overwhelming at times. It's full of daily duties and responsibilities and commitments. Work, appointments, childcare, and other activities can leave us frazzled. Yet when you're also dealing with chronic pain and illness, it doesn't take much to tip the scales. One additional task can increase pain and possibly cause panic to set in. It may even be hard to settle your mind and take a moment to just breathe.

David wrote today's verse, and he knew all about the ups and downs of life. He also knew that he could turn to God, cry out to Him, and trust that he would be heard. We can, and should, do the same. The Lord is our Refuge and our Comforter. He will guide us and give us strength to get through the most pressing tasks, such as getting out of bed, getting dressed, and eating. He will also offer us His peace, if we choose to accept it.

God is able to do above and beyond anything we ask or even consider asking. He will provide the strength needed to get through any situation. We were not created to be overwhelmed by trying to do life alone. When we shift our focus to God, it allows us to put everything in perspective. The Lord will even help us learn to say no to tasks that weigh us down and increase our stress load. So, when you notice the waves of pain and overload crashing in, don't feel that you need to do it all on your own. Look to God to lift you up. Use His shelter for prayer, as well as thanksgiving and praise. Accept the comfort He offers.

Lord, help me to turn to You first and accept the peace and comfort You,
my Refuge, are handing to me today. Amen.

Reflection

What is one task you can delegate to someone else so you can have time to breathe today?

_____

_____

_____

_____

_____

_____

_____

_____

_____

_____

_____

_____

_____

DAY 9

Fear

Don't worry about anything; instead, pray about everything.
Tell God what you need, and thank him for all he has done.

—Philippians 4:6

This has always been one of my favorite verses. In fact, many of my favorite verses have a similar theme: do not worry; do not fear; or do not be anxious. Ironically, I have a hard time following God's commands in these passages. I often wonder why that is—why it's so easy for me to give in to my fears and allow them to run wild in my mind.

My pastor told me this acronym for "fear" a few years ago, and I loved it: False Evidence Appearing Real. I have found it to be a powerful reminder that the majority of my anxieties never come to pass. The enemy, however, likes to blow things out of proportion every chance he gets. My symptoms and pain can be unpredictable, and chronic illness itself fuels fears. So, when the icepick stab, spasm, or a new symptom appears, the enemy grabs on to that and doesn't want to let go.

Worry is a powerful force, and it's prevalent in our society. Worry erodes the spirit and increases frustration, as well as pain. It can literally make us sick. And, sadly, it's not something we can totally eliminate on our own. That's where Philippians 4:6 comes into play.

Paul wrote today's verse. His words are an encouragement that while life is full of uncertainties and trials, God's faithfulness and love are always certain. Nothing is too big or too small to take to the Lord in prayer. In fact, His Word points out on numerous occasions that we are to cast our cares on Him. God offers us a peace beyond all understanding (Phil. 4:7). So, take your anxieties to Him in prayer today. Accept His peace. Then praise Him in advance for the promises He is working on your behalf.

> *Lord, thank You that I can come to You with anything*
> *and receive Your peace in return. Amen.*

Reflection

What will you release to God today?

_____

_____

_____

_____

_____

_____

_____

_____

_____

_____

_____

_____

DAY 10

God's in Control

*"So don't worry about tomorrow, for tomorrow will bring its own worries.
Today's trouble is enough for today."*

—Matthew 6:34

I woke up in the middle of the night with some alarming new symptoms. Of course, my mind jumped to the worst-case scenario—chest pain, so it must be a heart attack. To be safe, I woke up my husband, and we headed to the emergency room. The doctors concluded I had costochondritis, which is common with fibromyalgia. Costochondritis is inflammation of the cartilage that connects a rib to the sternum, and the pain it causes can mimic a heart condition. Upon explanation, I praised the Lord that it wasn't anything serious. Sadly, this was the beginning of many similar bouts—and a few trips to the hospital—with costochondritis, each one sending a wave of panic through my body and mind. Over the years, I've learned to recognize the signs, often in advance, but that doesn't mean I never jump to the worst conclusion possible.

Fear and worry are insidious. Sadly, they're a common occurrence for those battling chronic pain and illness. The cumulative effect wreaks havoc on our already-battered bodies and minds. The enemy knows our weaknesses, and he does what he can to ignite anxiety whenever possible. It's easy for him to do, as there are numerous things in life, particularly with pain and our bodies, that cause anxiety. Our minds can become stuck in the vicious cycle of what-if statements. Fear can take root and consume us. When we get anxious about things that may or may not happen, the only solution is to turn it all over to the Lord. He can replace those worries with His peace.

The best remedy for fear is to stop it before it begins to cycle. When fear and worry surface, speak to them. "I'm not going to let fear consume me." Then, instead of letting your thoughts go into overdrive, take your concerns to the Lord in prayer. Fear increases when our minds focus on the enemy's lies. Faith blooms when we meditate on God's Word. People dealing with chronic pain and illness already have a limited energy supply. Don't waste that energy on lies. Use your energy to build up your faith.

Lord, when fears and worries threaten to overtake me,
remind me to keep my focus on You. Amen.

Reflection

What unnecessary fears can you set aside today?

_____

_____

_____

_____

_____

_____

_____

_____

_____

DAY 11

Unchanging

Jesus Christ is the same yesterday, today, and forever.

—Hebrews 13:8

Life can change in an instant. I've heard people say that time and time again. However, I never truly knew the meaning behind that statement until 1994. On October 26, I learned just how accurate the comment was. That was the day I was hit by a car. The day a cop told me others had died at that very spot. The day my battle with chronic pain and illness began.

I've never been a fan of change. I like things to be predictable, comfortable even. That was no longer the case after October 26, 1994. My new "normal" forced me to make even more changes—just to do simple, everyday activities. No need to worry about being spontaneous. It's just not possible anymore. I never know if today is the day for a flare-up in my pain or fatigue, resulting in major adjustments to my schedule. That's not easy for someone who loves their to-do list!

After my accident, I couldn't just put my head in the sand and do nothing. I had to learn to adapt. Yet despite the pain, uncertainty, and fear I was experiencing—and still am—one thing didn't change: Jesus! And that's powerful! No matter what is happening in and around us, Jesus stays the same. Always. As Hebrews 13:8 reminds us, "Jesus Christ is the same yesterday, today, and forever." Present tense. Many things in life are ever-changing, especially with chronic pain. That can be scary and uncomfortable. Don't focus on what's shifting and beyond your control. Don't worry about the to-do list that may not get done until tomorrow. Focus on the One Who is always the same, the One constant we can always trust and depend on—Jesus.

Lord, thank You for the reminder that You don't change,
so I can find my strength, security, and peace in You. Amen.

Reflection

How can you alter the way you handle change?

_____

_____

_____

_____

_____

_____

_____

_____

_____

_____

_____

_____

_____

_____

DAY 12

He Knows Your Name

What is the price of five sparrows—two copper coins? Yet God does not forget
a single one of them. And the very hairs on your head are all numbered.
So don't be afraid; you are more valuable to God than a whole flock of sparrows.

—Luke 12:6-7

It took years for me to understand that sharing my story—including the pain, anxiety, and frustration—could be helpful, and perhaps healing, to others and, in turn, to me. For so long, I kept things hidden inside. I didn't want to be viewed as different. I didn't want them to see me as weak. Slowly, I came to a realization. The things I hated about myself for years were the very things God wanted to use. They weren't there to diminish me. They were there to make me stronger through Him.

Today's verse mentions sparrows. In general, birds are plentiful, thus easily overlooked. Matthew mentioned how two sparrows were sold for one penny. In Luke 12:6-7, he is saying that if you were to buy four, the fifth sparrow would be thrown in for free, essentially making it worthless in the eyes of many. However, that sparrow is not invaluable to or passed over by our heavenly Father. He cares about each and every one of them—just like He cares about each and every person.

Have you ever felt common, damaged, misunderstood, or overlooked? If so, know that it's not how God sees you. He made you unique. He sees you as His beloved. He values you. He knows you by name. You are made in His likeness. He knows every detail about you. He knows your struggles and insecurities. And He loves you just as you are! You are more than your pain, illness, anxiety, doubts, and fears. You are a beloved child of God. Psalm 139:2-3 states, "You know when I sit down or stand up. You know my thoughts even when I'm far away. You see me when I travel and when I rest at home. You know everything I do." Remember that the next time you are tempted to feel less than someone else. Rest assured that God sees you. He knows you. He loves you, just as you are.

Lord, help me to go forth today with my head held high knowing
that I am priceless to You. Amen.

Reflection

How does knowing how God feels about you change how you feel about yourself?

_____

_____

_____

_____

_____

_____

_____

_____

_____

_____

DAY 13

Silencing the Lies

And now, dear brothers and sisters, one final thing. Fix your thoughts on what is true, and honorable, and right, and pure, and lovely, and admirable. Think about things that are excellent and worthy of praise.

—Philippians 4:8

Why are you napping? Don't you have work to do? What about the dishes and laundry? And that lunch you promised your friend after stopping at the post office? You don't have time to take a break. You have too much to do today.

So much noise—not external, but in my head. The enemy slings condemning thoughts my way all day long. Some days, I'm great about taking them and turning them into a praise or prayer. But on the bad days—the days when it's a struggle to do the simplest task? Sadly, the devil gets a hold and doesn't let up easily. I may need to enlist my husband or a friend to help in the battle to shift my mind to God's still, small voice. *You know that isn't the truth. Don't listen to the lies. Fix your eyes on Me. I will give you rest. Let Me be your Strength.*

Paul is encouraging us in this verse to fix our thoughts on what is true, and honorable, and right, and pure, and lovely, and admirable. In doing so, we can erase the lies the enemy tries to make us believe about ourselves. God knows our weaknesses and struggles. He will not denounce us. He will show us the truth: that we are still—and always will be—His beloved, whether or not the dishes are washed or the clothes are put away. Choose to redirect your focus when you are tempted to get down on yourself. It can be easy to be pessimistic, especially when you are in pain. Instead of listening to the enemy's lies, replace the negative thoughts with positive notions, such as meditating on God's Word and filling your mind with praise and God's truths.

Lord, erase the lies that enter my mind and destroy my peace and help me focus instead on You. Amen.

Reflection

What lies can you dispel today?

_____

_____

_____

_____

_____

_____

_____

_____

_____

_____

_____

_____

_____

DAY 14

Not Alone

I pray that from his glorious, unlimited resources he will empower you with inner strength through his Spirit.

—Ephesians 3:16

I strive to come across as happy and put-together to others. However, in reality, I deal with chronic pain on a daily basis. Others can't see it, so they don't know what a struggle it is to appear strong—as though nothing is wrong, everything is normal, and I have it all under control. Let me be the first to say that the façade couldn't be further from the truth most days.

I'll admit that it's not my own strength that gets me through each day. My plans are often derailed by a stabbing headache, fatigue, or muscle spasms. On those days, it's quite obvious that my strength comes from the Lord. I learned a long time ago that I can't do it all on my own, and neither can you. The good news is that we weren't meant to do life—including all its struggles—without help.

We all have weaknesses we can't escape, ones that are beyond human strength. Paul reminds us in Ephesians 3:16 that it's okay to need help. It's not weakness to ask for assistance. Paul was a spiritual giant, yet he went through trying times where he realized he couldn't handle it all on his own. He turned to Jesus, and we can do the same. Our strength is limited, but the Lord's isn't. As the verse states, He has "unlimited resources." In weakness, His power can shine through. His Spirit is living inside of you. It's a gift, and you are not an exception to that precious gift. By drinking from the fountain (His Word), you can have all you need to get through any situation you may encounter. So run to Him. Cast your cares on Him (1 Peter 5:7). Feel His strength inside of you. You are a child of God. He will encourage you and meet you right where you are.

Lord, thank You that Your grace is all I need. Amen.

Reflection

Where can God be strong in your weakness?

_____

_____

_____

_____

_____

_____

_____

_____

_____

_____

_____

_____

_____

_____

DAY 15

Perfect Peace

You will keep in perfect peace all who trust in you,
all whose thoughts are fixed on you!

—Isaiah 26:3

No matter who we are or where we are in our journeys, everybody needs a little patience—and sometimes a lot of patience—with others and ourselves. If you are a chronic pain or chronic illness warrior, that statement is even truer. Whether it's waiting for a joyful event, such as graduation or a vacation, or waiting for a flare-up to pass, patience is required.

Patience doesn't come naturally for me, even on a good day. As a Type A personality, my stress level is quite high. I have daily to-do lists, and I try my best to keep things going according to my plan. Yet when widespread pain is thrown in, that stress level climbs beyond measure. "Perfect peace" is nowhere to be found—especially in my overactive mind. Unless someone is also battling chronic pain and illness, the challenge is not something most people understand, so that necessitates additional patience when dealing with others—in addition to the patience we must offer ourselves.

God gave the prophet Isaiah an amazing promise—He "will keep [you] in perfect peace." That promise applies to us, too! But in order to have it, our minds must stay fixed on the Lord. Doing so can take practice. The enemy will use our pain to try and distract us. He wants us to forget the One Who is our Strength, our Hope, and our Peace. I've found that if I take a few moments to be alone, breathe deeply, and refocus my thoughts by placing them on the Lord, I can feel a sense of His peace—the "peace, which exceeds anything we can understand" (Phil. 4:7). While it doesn't automatically fix everything or make me pain-free, it does help me remember that God is still in control. Peace and patience can always be found by resting in Him.

Lord, when my patience is running low and my pain and stress high,
help me to place my focus on You and accept Your perfect peace. Amen.

Reflection

In what area can God's perfect peace help you have a little more patience today?

_____

_____

_____

_____

_____

_____

_____

_____

_____

_____

_____

_____

DAY 16

One Day at a Time

Your Father already knows your needs. Seek the Kingdom of God above all else, and he will give you everything you need.

—Luke 12:30-31

I sighed as the alarm went off. I hadn't slept more than an hour all night due to the pain. Instead, I tossed and turned and watched the clock. And now, I had a migraine on top of everything else. It was a struggle just to get out of bed and dressed. I'm already dreading the day as I mentally run through my to-do list and head out the door. I'd love to stay in bed, but my body hurts too much to even do that.

Mornings like this are rough. On those days, planned activities may not get done. When this happens, there's one thing on my schedule that's more important than anything else, even if nothing else gets crossed off my list. It's something I do each morning—my daily devotional time with the Lord. That is when I spend time reading His Word and praying. I also turn my to-do list over to Him so He can prioritize my day.

We can choose to fixate on our circumstances, such as our pain, or we can fixate on the One Who already knows our needs, the One Who can give us strength to get through whatever we encounter. It's a choice that must be made on a daily basis. When you seek God first, He will give you the strength you need each day to do what you need to do . . . even if it's not everything you have planned. When you're battling fatigue and pain on a daily—or even hourly—basis, your job is to look to Him and take things one moment at a time. One breath at a time. He knows what you require to get through the day.

Lord, I don't need to worry about my to-do list because I know You'll give me the strength I need in order to do all You ask of me. Amen.

Reflection

What is the most important thing God needs you to do today?

_____

_____

_____

_____

_____

_____

_____

_____

_____

_____

_____

_____

_____

DAY 17

Rest in Jesus

Then Jesus said, "Come to me, all of you who are weary and carry heavy burdens,
and I will give you rest."

—Matthew 11:28

Rest. Wow! What a concept. It often eludes me, so what Matthew mentions in this verse is hard to fathom, yet it is also appealing. It's something I long for. I was brought up with the mindset that I should always be doing something. I come from a hardworking farm family. There was little downtime because there were always chores to be done.

The need to keep busy has stuck with me all my life, especially after I heard someone say that "idle hands are the devil's playthings." However, my body doesn't always want to cooperate. Fatigue and pain tell me I need to rest on occasion, and it's usually at the most inconvenient times. But if and when I do sit down and try to rest my body, my mind still runs, thinking of everything I should be doing instead. My brain is like a computer with way too many windows and tabs open. I also worry that others are judging me. I envision them speculating on why I'm not doing something—anything but sitting down. Perhaps you can relate.

For those with chronic pain, weariness is a familiar and common occurrence. Jesus said in today's passage that He will give us rest. That means it's okay to do nothing—to just be—with our body and mind. Jesus does not want us to be overwhelmed, overburdened, or overworked.

Jesus's offer is simple yet profound. He is the Solution to every challenge we face. That promise can lift whatever weighs us down. As it states in Matthew 11:28, the Lord will give us rest. So today, set aside a few minutes to be still and take some deep breaths. Invite the Lord into your day. Allow your body and mind to accept and embrace the peace and rest Jesus is offering.

Lord, I will take time today to blow out my anxiety
and breathe in Your peace as I rest in You. Amen.

Reflection

How can you find ways to rest your body and mind today?

_____

_____

_____

_____

_____

_____

_____

_____

_____

_____

_____

_____

_____

DAY 18

Strength in Stillness

Wait patiently for the LORD. Be brave and courageous.
Yes, wait patiently for the Lord.

—Psalm 27:14

I remember my gram singing a song to me as a child about the importance of being patient. Apparently, my drive to be on the go started early on, along with my lack of patience and difficulty waiting. Sadly, that's followed me around all my life.

My mind's "need" to keep going and my "inability" to sit still and wait patiently are in sharp contrast to what my chronic pain and illness tell me. I assume others are thinking the same thoughts I tell myself. *Why are you just sitting there? I know you have stuff you need to do. Get going!*

David tells us to wait patiently for the Lord. A lot of waiting is involved with chronic illness, from obtaining a diagnosis to specialist appointments to finding an effective treatment. *But, Lord, I want to be healed now. I've been waiting for over twenty-five years. When will my healing come?* Sound familiar?

When I look back, I can see that God has always been there. He's gotten me through days I thought were too much to bear. He held me up when I wanted to give in. My inability to wait patiently didn't make Him move any faster. However, He redirected me and gave me hope when I thought there was none. He gave me patience and strength to face another day.

The Bible is full of "waiters." Noah waited eight months to get off the ark. David spent fourteen years fleeing Saul before David became king. And Abraham was one hundred years old before he had a son. We are called to "search for the LORD and for his strength; continually seek him" (1 Chron. 16:11). God knows our illness. He understands our limitations and is there with us, even in our pain. Cling to Him. Wait patiently on Him to guide you and show you His plan for your life.

Lord, forgive my impatience when I want things to go according to my timetable instead of Yours. Amen.

Reflection

What challenges do you face in being still and waiting patiently on the Lord?

_____

_____

_____

_____

_____

_____

_____

_____

_____

_____

_____

DAY 19

A Purpose for the Pain

And we know that God causes everything to work together for the good of those who love God and are called according to his purpose for them.

—Romans 8:28

Ten long years. That's how long it took for me to finally have a name for what I'd been living with for so long. Countless doctor appointments and tests. Feeling like everything was all in my mind. Being told the results were "normal" and there was nothing wrong with me. However, I knew my body, and I was certain the doctors were wrong. The fatigue and pain were different and more widespread than anything I'd ever experienced. Finally, I had a name—fibromyalgia. I literally hugged the physician's assistant when she gave me the diagnosis. Someone had actually listened to me and looked over my extensive, growing list of symptoms. Most importantly, *she believed me!*

I was elated that I finally knew what was going on with me, but I was also devastated. I grieved the loss of the "me" I'd once been and would likely never be again. I felt broken and alone. None of my friends or loved ones could even begin to grasp what I was going through.

Fibromyalgia is one of many invisible illnesses. That means that, often, sufferers look fine on the outside, though that's not how they feel on the inside. Their lives have changed in dramatic ways.

In Romans 8:28, Paul isn't telling us that pain and suffering are good or pleasant. They're not. Instead, he is reminding us that we can be confident

God will never desert us. He has a plan for us. This is a certainty we know. Job struggled and endured much pain. Yet he told the Lord, "'I know that you can do anything, and no one can stop you'" (Job 42:2). This new "normal" you're living is a reminder that, as a Christ-follower, you will still have troubles and trials, but you won't go through them alone. God is with you. He cares about you. He will provide for your needs. He has a purpose for each ache and pain you experience. Nothing is wasted with Him.

Lord, help me to trust that You use everything for Your good
and that my illness is an opportunity to draw closer to You. Amen.

Reflection

How did God comfort you when you received your diagnosis?

_____

_____

_____

_____

_____

_____

_____

_____

_____

_____

_____

DAY 20

In Christ Alone

For I can do everything through Christ, who gives me strength.

—Philippians 4:13

I don't know why, but I often feel like I have to do everything on my own. Somewhere along the way, it became stuck in my mind that that's the way it's supposed to be. I hate asking for help from anyone, including loved ones and even God.

I have always worried about what others think about me. Do they view me differently because I have chronic pain and illness? Asking for help seems like an admittance of weakness. I try my best to put up a strong front, so others don't realize I'm struggling or in pain. Of course, by overextending myself, my pain increases. I paste on a smile and power through, no matter what. My mind constantly runs through to-do lists and all the possible options, and I often feel overwhelmed. But I'm an adult, so I should be able to do it all by myself. Right? Wrong.

We're human, so struggles are inevitable. However, they are also a chance to ask for assistance. (Yes, it's really okay to do that!) Challenges are an opportunity to reach out to God for help, to draw close to Him. He didn't design us to get through life on our own. He wants us to ask for help (1 John 5:14-15), and He will be there to help us.

The apostle Paul wrote Philippians 4:13 in a prison cell. Through all the dismal conditions, Paul knew he had the strength to endure. Paul was certain of this because he had a relationship with Jesus. As a result of that, Paul was confident that he could face anything and would never be alone. Christ-followers have that same assurance. There is no point in being upset about the things you can't do. Your pain and illness are no surprise to God. Turn to the Lord. He will provide the armor needed for any battle you face.

Lord, help me to prioritize my day and find the balance between productivity and peace, which can only be obtained through You. Amen.

Reflection

What do you need help with today?

_____

_____

_____

_____

_____

_____

_____

_____

_____

_____

_____

_____

_____

DAY 21

Preparing for Battle

You have armed me with strength for the battle.

—Psalm 18:39

Dealing with chronic pain is tough. It is quite literally a pain, in every sense of the word. I've told my husband on many occasions that I'm pretty sure my pain is determined to hit every single body part. Some days, doing a basic task, such as showering or getting dressed, can be a struggle. That one activity may end up being the only thing you do in a day. And if so, that's okay. No matter what you do or don't do, you are still a child of God.

God knows that life will be difficult at times. You won't be able to handle everything on your own. The wonderful news is that you do not have to go through it alone (Deut. 31:6). He is there to help you, but you have to let Him do so. Call out to Him, and He will give you the strength you need for battle—even if that battle is your basic daily routine or one within your own body.

Psalm 18 was written by David. It's about deliverance and protection. When clothed with God's power, David was able to defeat his enemies. Though our enemy—pain—is different, we, too, can do the same. As David mentions in verse nineteen, "He rescued me because He delights in me." Here's some wonderful news: God delights in us, too!

God is good. He is on your side, and He has a purpose for every pain you are dealing with today. With each stab, throb, or spasm, go to the Lord. Let Him assist you. As it states in Isaiah 40:29, "He gives power to the weak and strength to the powerless." When you ask God for help, He will give you what you need to face each day—one day at a time, one moment at a time. You may not develop superhero strength, but God will provide all you need.

Lord, thank You for equipping me for each battle I face,
whether it's within my body or external, each and every day. Amen.

Reflection

What battle can God help you with today?

_____

_____

_____

_____

_____

_____

_____

_____

_____

_____

_____

_____

_____

_____

DAY 22

Finding Refreshment in the Lord

Then times of refreshment will come from the presence of the Lord,
and he will again send you Jesus, your appointed Messiah.

—Acts 3:20

People find refreshment in a variety of ways—an invigorating walk in nature, a cold glass of lemonade, a relaxing bubble bath, or a comfy chair and a good book. While these activities could be enjoyable for many people, the same things may not work as well for someone dealing with chronic pain and illness. What is enjoyable one day could be agonizing the next. It's a fine line, and it's often paved with many trials and errors.

There is one thing, however, that can bring refreshment to anyone, no matter the level of pain that day—pausing to spend time with the Lord. This could come in the form of His Word, worship music, or just taking a moment to be still and listen to what He wants to say to you, His precious daughter. He is called "the bread of life" (John 6:35). Merely spending time in His presence is refreshing, to the mind, body, and spirit.

I find that on my good days, it's hard for me to take a moment to "just be." I like to get in as much work as I can on those days to try and balance out the bad days. However, I often realize that I get a gentle nudge, and that causes me to stop. If I'm too busy to pause for God, I'm too busy in general. Whether it's a short prayer of thanks or a plea to get through the day, time spent with the Lord will always be rewarded with His peace.

Lord, as I go through my day today, help me remember to pause for a moment
of peace that can come only from spending time with You. Amen.

Reflection

When can you take a moment to pause today and spend time with the Lord?

_____

_____

_____

_____

_____

_____

_____

_____

_____

_____

_____

_____

_____

_____

_____

_____

DAY 23

Unanswered Prayers

Father, if you are willing, please take this cup of suffering away from me.
Yet I want your will to be done, not mine.

—Luke 22:42

One of my favorite songs by country music star Garth Brooks is "Unanswered Prayers," where he thanks God for the silly, youthful prayers that never came to pass—specifically in relation to his high school girlfriend who didn't become his wife. When I was a teenager, I had similar prayers. *If only he would look my way, everything would be perfect.* However, by the time I entered college, I was doing what Garth did—thanking God that He knew what He was doing when He didn't answer my prayers the way I thought He should.

Since my accident in 1994, my prayers have changed. I've spent countless hours praying for God to heal me and take away the pain I've experienced every single day for over twenty-five years. Granted, some days are better than others, but the pain is always there. Some days, it's difficult to submit to God's will, accepting that He has a plan. I have questioned at times why I'm not one He chooses to heal, like I've seen Him do for others. I've also wondered if He is even listening to me. Perhaps you've wondered the same thing.

It's easy and natural to question and even feel disappointed when we're in pain. We may not always understand why God does what He does, but it's important to remember what Luke said in today's verse—particularly the ending: "Yet I want your will to be done, not mine." He may not always deliver us from a situation, but we can be confident that He will provide grace and strength to endure. Jesus struggled with God's will, but He knew that His Father saw the larger picture. We, too, can trust that God knows what He's doing, even with our unanswered prayers.

Lord, I know You only want what's best for me, even when I don't understand, and I'm choosing to trust You. Amen.

Reflection

What prayers can you trust God with today?

_____

_____

_____

_____

_____

_____

_____

_____

_____

_____

_____

_____

_____

DAY 24

As Sweet as Honey

Kind words are like honey—sweet to the soul and healthy for the body.

—Proverbs 16:24

Have you ever had someone pay you a compliment? Do you remember how it made you feel? Odds are it made you feel good about yourself—happy, even. And if you were having a bad day prior to that comment, it may have even turned around the remainder of your day.

Now, take a moment to listen to what you're saying to yourself. What do you hear? Are the messages things you'd tell your friends or loved ones? Are they positive and life-affirming? Or are the words negative and condemning? If what you're saying isn't something you would tell someone you care about, then why are you thinking them about yourself? Perhaps you've heard people say, "If you don't have anything nice to say, then don't say anything." Well, there is a lot of truth to that statement, even when you're speaking to yourself.

It's easy to get down on yourself, especially when dealing with chronic pain and illness. You may be frustrated that your body isn't cooperating and letting you do what your mind wants to do. But it's important to remember that words hold a great amount of power. They shape us. They can be honey (today's verse) or poison (James 3:7-8). Words can increase our stress level and pain, or they can cause us to momentarily focus on something else. Just because you're having a bad day or not accomplishing all you hoped to do today doesn't mean you're a failure. You're alive, and God is a God of second, third, and even one hundred chances. Tomorrow is a new day. Take a moment right now to speak life-giving words over yourself. Be thankful and praise God for what you were able to do today. You woke up. You're reading this. What else can you add to the list? Focus on those accomplishments instead of the things you didn't do. Set your mind on the positives and speak helpful, soothing words to yourself.

Lord, make my self-talk as sweet as honey and allow me to hear what You have to say to me today. Amen.

Reflection

What can you praise God for today?

_____

_____

_____

_____

_____

_____

_____

_____

_____

_____

_____

_____

DAY 25

Jesus Understands

Turn to me and have mercy, for I am alone and in deep distress.

—Psalm 25:16

I'm self-employed, so I spend a lot of time alone. I don't have many nearby friends who deal with chronic pain and illness. Most of the people who truly understand are friends I've met online. Therefore, my struggles can make me feel lonely sometimes. For the majority of the day, it's just me and my turtle. As much as I love him, he's not concerned about whether or not I need assistance or worried about if I am having a good day. He doesn't hear me cry out when I'm in pain.

My husband is extremely patient and quite helpful when he's with me. He is understanding. But like my other friends and family members, he doesn't truly feel what I'm going through. He may see that I'm not feeling well or having problems completing a task, but he can't fully experience my struggle. In fact, few people in my day-to-day life truly comprehend what I'm experiencing.

Loneliness often accompanies illness. Sure, we need time alone to rest and recover. However, many with chronic pain or illness push others—including loved ones and God—away, often unintentionally.

Jesus understands loneliness. He stepped away from His disciples when they left Him in the Garden of Gethsemane. Jesus would also withdraw to spend time with God and be strengthened (John 16:32). He saw being alone as a gift—a time to get closer to His Father and draw from His strength—and it can be the same for us.

Our faith can blossom in the desert times as we draw closer to God. David was hemmed in by troubles all around him. He was being pursued by Saul, and he had no idea whom he could trust. Yet David knew the Lord was there for him. Those times were rich with spiritual growth for David. Our difficult times can be for us, as well. We're never left alone, wandering in the desert. Though we may not always feel Him, we can be confident that the Lord is always walking beside us.

Lord, thank You for never leaving me alone and for using the desert times as a chance to draw me closer to You. Amen.

Reflection

What can you learn in your desert time with God?

_____

_____

_____

_____

_____

_____

_____

_____

_____

_____

DAY 26

Unrealistic Expectations

We all make many mistakes.

—James 3:2

I'm a perfectionist—or at least my mind strives to be one. Logically, I know it's unrealistic. However, I still push myself to do my best, not make a mistake, and control every situation down to the tiniest detail in just about everything I do. I hold myself to high standards that are impossible to attain. And even when I do meet my own standards, it comes at the expense of extra pressure. That pressure to be perfect adds to my stress, which adds to my pain, which adds to my frustration, which adds to my—you name it. There is always something to worry about, some (often unrealistic) goal to strive toward. It's a vicious cycle—one that ultimately leads to self-destruction.

Does any of this sound familiar to you? If so, let me share some advice I was given recently—stop beating yourself up. It's okay to stumble or be less than perfect. *No one* on earth is perfect. And that's okay, because God loves you *just as you are.*

Perfectionism may seem harmless on the surface. It is always a good idea to try and do your best when possible—but not at the expense of causing increased pain and stress. The realization that we aren't perfect reinforces our need for Christ. Allow yourself to relinquish control, take a breath, and enjoy the moment. If you stumble and fall in your endeavors—and you will at some point—don't worry. Don't be hard on yourself. It doesn't mean you've failed or that you're a failure. It means you're human. God will pick you up, plant your feet on solid ground, and give you multiple chances to try again. His grace and mercy are new each and every day.

Lord, deliver me from my perceived need for perfection, as the only perfect One is Jesus, and Your opinion is the only one that matters. Amen.

Reflection

What perceived need can you release to the Lord today?

_____

_____

_____

_____

_____

_____

_____

_____

_____

_____

_____

_____

_____

_____

_____

_____

Change the Channel

Always be joyful. Never stop praying. Be thankful in all circumstances,
for this is God's will for you who belong to Christ Jesus.

—1 Thessalonians 5:16-18

Many people spend a lot of time thinking about what they don't have, what they don't like about themselves, and who they wish they were. I know I've often focused on the tiny dot in the center of a big sheet of paper—the little annoyances versus the blessings, the momentary pain instead of life's joys.

I'm reminded of a story I heard from a teaching colleague years ago. One of her students couldn't wait to tell her about his new glasses. She assumed he was happy about them because he could finally see the board. But that wasn't the case. He was excited because he was sure that girls wouldn't want to kiss him if he had glasses on. (He was in the second grade!) What a great reminder! It's all about perspective.

It's okay to be upset and grieve the fact that you may not be where you thought you'd be at this stage in life. The shortest verse in the Bible reminds us that Jesus wasn't always joyful either (John 11:35). You have to remember you're a work in progress, and with God's help, anything is possible. Perhaps you don't have the perfect life you dreamed you'd have, but you are alive—and that is a tremendous blessing. There is no time like the present to reframe your focus. Our minds are like TV stations—there are hundreds of options to choose from. Don't get stuck on the negative ones. Change the channel! Notice the blessings God has placed in your life. Choose to praise Him when you feel like getting down on yourself. Send up prayers instead of worrying about the new symptom or flare-up that occurred today. Believe that God has great plans for you because He *can* and *will* use you as you are, right where you are.

Lord, thank You for the many blessings in my life and for being a good and generous God. Amen.

Reflection

What channel do you need to turn off today?

_____

_____

_____

_____

_____

_____

_____

_____

_____

_____

_____

_____

_____

DAY 28

Perseverance

But as for you, be strong and courageous, for your work will be rewarded.

—2 Chronicles 15:7

If you are dealing with chronic pain and illness, you know how easy it is to get down on yourself, feel frustrated, and lose faith. It almost becomes second nature to get discouraged and focus on what you can't do. This is particularly true on days when things don't go as planned. You see little progress on projects you've been trying to finish for days. You compare yourself to others who appear to have it all together. Or it may even feel like you're moving two steps backward instead of forward. It's hard, at times, to believe there's a light at the end of the proverbial tunnel.

In 2 Chronicles 15:7, Azariah, Obed's son, was speaking to King Asa. The leaders had been ready to give up, but King Asa's perspective changed. He stayed committed to the Lord and didn't give up. He persevered.

It's important not to let your limitations discourage you. Life's circumstances do not dictate your joy. Remember Azariah's words and stay encouraged. Keep your focus upward versus inward and take heart. God's not finished with you yet. In fact, He's using these moments to help you grow into the person He created you to be.

God sees you. Don't forget that. Even when you feel invisible or like you're stuck on the hamster wheel of life, He sees you. He is with you. He loves you. Set aside a moment to listen to God today. Hear His still, small voice encouraging you to be strong in Him and to not give up. He will fill you with the perseverance to get through the day—to do what you need to do, what you hope to do, and what He's calling you to do. He will use you right where you are.

Lord, thank You for propping me up and helping me persevere
when I feel like giving up. Amen.

Reflection

How is God encouraging you today?

_____

_____

_____

_____

_____

_____

_____

_____

_____

_____

_____

_____

_____

DAY 29

Dream Big

Not that I was ever in need, for I have learned how to be content with whatever I have. I know how to live on almost nothing or with everything. I have learned the secret of living in every situation, whether it is with a full stomach or empty, with plenty or little.

—Philippians 4:11-12

As a little girl, I dreamed of the future. I had so many grand plans, as I'm sure many people do. However, being hit by a car a few months prior to getting married was not on my life's to-do list. While a doctor told me almost immediately that I'd have arthritis as a result of my injuries, it took close to a year before my symptoms snowballed. I realized there was more going on than just arthritis. Daily pain and fatigue became commonplace, and I had no idea why. The only thing I knew was that I could no longer envision what my future held.

Ten years later, I was given my first official diagnosis—fibromyalgia. I experienced a roller coaster of emotions and thoughts. I was upset and frustrated. I felt broken. I wanted things to be how they used to be. Chronic pain and illness were not something my husband or I had signed up for.

Paul knew about the "good old days." Yet he learned to be content. He realized that true contentment isn't found in life's circumstances. It's only found in Jesus, the One Who gave Paul strength to get through every situation. And the Lord can do the same for us.

There's no such thing as a trouble-free life. Pain and adversity are inevitable. Yet they're not an automatic cause to panic and give our mind and power over to the enemy. Setbacks can steal our joy, but only if we allow it to happen. It takes work to come to terms with a new "normal." Yet over time, it's possible to replace some of the "what-could've-beens" with trust in the Lord. Continue to dream big. God has plans for you, and He is enough for everything you'll encounter in life.

Lord, thank You that You will meet my every need
and I can find true contentment in You alone. Amen.

Reflection

What "could've-beens" can you set aside in order to be more content in the life the Lord has lined up for you?

DAY 30

Life's Storms

If we are thrown into the blazing furnace, the God whom we serve is able to save us.

—Daniel 3:17

Life is full of storms right now. It can be hard to keep the faith at times. Things like hate and violence are everywhere in the world, making it feel like a dangerous place to live. If you're dealing with chronic pain and illness, some of those storms are occurring inside your body, and that can be scary. It's hard not to let fears and anxieties run amuck, especially when your pain and illness seem to have a mind of their own. But through it all, God is still God.

Shadrach, Meshach, and Abednego placed their confidence in God. These three Hebrew men were thrown into a fiery furnace by Nebuchadnezzar, the king of Babylon, because they refused to bow down to the king's image. They were faced with a dire situation, but their faith in God never faltered. During their trials, God didn't abandoned them—and He hasn't abandoned you either. God is good. All the time. And He has plans for you.

No matter what is happening around—or even inside—us, God is still in control. I'm not saying you shouldn't watch the news and be informed or take notice of pain and flare-ups. You should. However, it's also not a good idea to take in too much and place all your focus on the passing storms. They're transient. With chronic pain and illness, many things that are occurring are likely beyond your control. Stressing about it will do little to change things or have a positive impact on the situation. Therefore, it is best to leave it all in God's very capable hands. Just as Jesus saved Shadrach, Meshach, and Abednego, He can save you and protect you from any "fires" in your life, mind, and body, as well.

Lord, I want the peace You offer when the storms of life seem out of control. Amen.

Reflection

What storms can you ask Jesus to calm for you today?

_____

_____

_____

_____

_____

_____

_____

_____

_____

_____

_____

_____

_____

_____

_____

DAY 31

A Thief Named Anxiety

I lie awake thinking of you, meditating on you through the night. Because you are my helper, I sing for joy in the shadow of your wings. I cling to you; your strong right hand holds me securely.

—Psalm 63:6-8

Again? Can't I have one night of sleep? One night where I don't toss and turn while he sleeps soundly? One night where my mind isn't trying to figure everything out?

Way too many nights go this way for me. Shooting pain in my back, hip, or shoulder makes me unable to find a comfortable position. I flip back and forth. My mind ruminates over the past day, week, and even year. Through it all, my husband sleeps peacefully, unaware of my struggle. Does this sound at all familiar to you?

I am anxious and in pain during the day, and both are often increased at night. There's nothing but silence to attempt to combat the swirling thoughts, anxiety, and widespread pain. There couldn't be a worse time to wrestle with things. In general, there's not much I can do about some things, such as my pain, during the day. There's even less I can do in the middle of the night.

At the time, it may feel like I'm alone battling my body to find rest. But that's not really the case. I'm never truly alone. Neither are you. Along with the pain and those racing thoughts, the Lord is there. Cry out to Him. Let Him take the weight off your shoulders. Look up. He's right there, waiting to offer comfort. "Come to me . . . and I will give you rest'" (Matt. 11:28).

Don't waste time going over and over in your mind what you should've done instead or could've done differently. You can't go back and change the past. However, there are things you can do. Pray. Recite worship song lyrics or Scripture verses. Let the Lord place a blanket over your worries and pain. Breathe in His peace.

Lord, thank You that I can cling to You at any time, and You will keep me safe and secure so I can rest in You. Amen.

Reflection

Which option will you use (prayer, song lyrics, or Scripture verse) to pull the Lord close when you can't sleep?

_____

_____

_____

_____

_____

_____

_____

_____

_____

_____

_____

_____

_____

DAY 32

Count It All Joy

Dear brothers and sisters, when troubles of any kind come your way,
consider it an opportunity for great joy.

—James 1:2

I was on a deadline, and I needed to work. But my body was telling me otherwise. Everything hurt, and I had a fever. My husband told me to "take it easy" and "just rest"—two phrases not typically found in my vocabulary. However, I felt so miserable that I reluctantly agreed. I listened to his advice, as well as my body. After a day of rest (and Netflix!), I felt better.

James is not saying I should have been happy because I was sick. Today's verse serves as a reminder that no matter how I feel, I can be joyful. My joy is not linked to my circumstances, and neither is yours.

For Christians, true joy is found in Jesus. Life is full of trials. Stress. Anxiety. Chronic illness. However, none of those things have to steal your joy. No amount of chaos is beyond God's control. James is a perfect example. He experienced numerous trials. His struggles increased his perseverance.

Life's challenges are given to help us grow and learn to trust. That day I was sick, I trusted my husband's advice, and my body thanked me for it. I endured and persevered and came out on the other side a few days later. My work was still there, and the world hadn't ended because I didn't get things finished a few days earlier.

Like our bodies need rest, so do our spirits and minds. Turn to God in trying times. Suffering and trials are designed to produce an unshakable faith. Trust in the Lord. Find your strength in Him. Allow Him to be your peace and comfort. Let the Lord be your joy in any and every situation.

Lord, help me to look to You when faced with trials
so I can stay strong and count it all joy. Amen.

Reflection

Do you listen to your body when it tells you it needs a rest?

_____

_____

_____

_____

_____

_____

_____

_____

_____

_____

_____

_____

_____

_____

DAY 33

Shift Your Perspective

And God will generously provide all you need. Then you will always have
everything you need and plenty left over to share with others.

—2 Corinthians 9:8

You had the day perfectly planned out, down to the most minute details. However, your plans didn't include having a flat tire, nearly unbearable pain, overwhelming fatigue, or some other unexpected event. Instead of smooth sailing, you watched your best-laid plans fly out the window before lunchtime.

It's all too easy to beat yourself up when life doesn't go as expected. We tend to focus on the small moments—on the *now* instead of the big picture. We aren't privy to the big picture, but God is. That's what He looks at.

Have you ever tried to change your perspective and focus on what you *did* accomplish during the day? You woke up. You showered. You got dressed. You ate breakfast. Perhaps you completed a number of other tasks, too. Maybe you considered all these activities as insignificant at the time. They're not. The most important thing about today is that you're alive! That's a huge blessing—a true gift from God.

Paul reminds us in 2 Corinthians 9:8 that "God will generously provide all that you need." His grace and mercy never end. He will bless you abundantly and meet *all* your needs, above and beyond any expectations you may have set for yourself. God's gifts do not depend on what we do or on what our pain prevents us from doing. You may not always have what you *want*, but God will give you what you *need* to get through the day or even the next moment. And everything—from the perfect day to perfect healing—will come in God's perfect timing. His resources and grace are unlimited.

Lord, I thank You that even when things don't go as planned, I'm alive,
and I know You will provide—today and every day. Amen.

Reflection

How can you shift your perspective today?

_____

_____

_____

_____

_____

_____

_____

_____

_____

_____

_____

_____

_____

_____

DAY 34

Life's Roller Coasters

In that day he will be your sure foundation, providing a rich store of salvation, wisdom, and knowledge.

—Isaiah 33:6

I've never been a fan of roller coasters. At the urging of some friends in high school, I reluctantly stood in line, waiting to ride one. By most people's standards, it would be considered a baby roller coaster—but it was more than big enough to terrify me. The other kids in line were jumping up and down, talking in great detail about various points of the ride. The more they discussed the ride, the more certain I was that I was making a huge mistake. And the more they witnessed my unease, the more animated and detailed their descriptions became! My group was up next, and I did get on the roller coaster. Thankfully, I survived. And that one ride was enough to let me know that I didn't want, or need, to do it again.

Ironically, since being diagnosed with multiple chronic illnesses, I often feel like I'm still on that ride—every single day. It's anything but fun for a person who likes life's events to be predictable, perhaps even boring, by some people's standards.

Life with chronic pain and chronic illness is a lot like that roller coaster. Just when you think things have finally leveled out and you have a handle on your symptoms, there's another ramp up or steep drop. Symptoms and pain come and go, to the point that you never know what to expect from one day to the next. And trying to jam everything into one of the "good days" is equally disastrous. It's challenging to make plans and experience life when you live with an illness full of symptoms that fluctuate multiple times a day. It is anything but stable. Thankfully, no matter where we may be on the chronic pain and illness roller coaster, our safety bar—God—is securely latched. He is our constant, and He will remain faithful through all the ups and downs.

Lord, thank You for being the One I can always rely on. Amen.

Reflection

Which of God's promises can you cling to when you're dealing with life's roller coasters?

_____

_____

_____

_____

_____

_____

_____

_____

_____

_____

_____

_____

DAY 35

God's Masterpiece

The Lord will work out his plans for my life—
for your faithful love, O Lord, endures forever.

—Psalm 138:8

We made pottery one year in art class when I was in elementary school. For a kid, it was a lot of fun. Messy, squishy, creative fun. We could make anything we wanted. Most students, including myself, decided to make a bowl. A few were a bit more adventurous, trying various animals. However, no matter what item was attempted, the result was still the same—nobody's object looked like they thought it would.

All the pieces had imperfections. Some didn't sit flat or were lumpy. Others were too skinny or too fat in one spot. Many of the "animals" looked like anything but an animal. Yet the teacher praised all of us. I'm sure the parents felt and responded the same way our teacher did when those misshapen items found their way home.

Each one of us is a bit like those pieces of imperfect, misshapen pottery. Our lives can be messy. Ideas may not turn out as hoped for or anticipated. Some things might be left unfinished. However, none of that matters to the Lord. He still has plans for each one of us.

God is the Master Artist. He knows we're still works in progress. We're unique. God did that for a reason. He will blend and shape us as He chooses until we are just perfect for His plans. He'll continue to mold us as long as we're here on earth. Pain, fatigue, and discouragement will never change that. Your pain and illness are not an accident. Our imperfections make us more like Christ. It's okay to be imperfect and unfinished. God finds beauty in our imperfection. Those scars cannot change His plans. We're still God's masterpieces.

Lord, thank You for using my imperfect life—and my illness—
to bring honor and glory to You. Amen.

Reflection

How have you seen God shape you over the past year?

_____

_____

_____

_____

_____

_____

_____

_____

_____

_____

_____

_____

_____

DAY 36

Finish the Race

I have fought the good fight, I have finished the race, and I have remained faithful.

—2 Timothy 4:7

I've never considered myself much of an athlete, and I don't enjoy running. Yet living with a chronic illness is very much like participating in a race. Athletes spend months training for events or games. Sadly, for chronic pain sufferers, we often are unaware of the fact that we even signed up to participate.

Physical *and* emotional training are required when dealing with chronic pain and illness. There are increased emotions when you're at the starting line, from the excitement of finally having a diagnosis to encouragement to finish strong. There's a plan and a set route to follow. However, some courses have unexpected obstacles and detours. Numerous trials and errors. Then doubts creep in, along with questions on whether it's possible to even finish the race.

When I received my first diagnosis over two decades ago, I thought things would go smoothly from there. After all, I finally had a name for what was happening. Unfortunately, I never imagined all the twists and turns that would occur along the way. Pacing is important. Sometimes, that will need to be adjusted on a regular basis. It's also imperative to establish priorities.

Today's verse was penned by the apostle Paul. He knew all about fighting the good fight. He found that the key is staying faithful to the Lord. That includes spending time with Him daily. There will be times when you feel God has given you more than you can handle. Before discounting that, take a look at all you've overcome to get to where you are today. You may have had to adjust your route along the way, but you've gained valuable coping skills. You've grown stronger in spirit and faith. The finish line is ahead of you. God is there, with His arms wide open, rooting you on. He will give you the strength to take one more step and finish strong.

Lord, help me stay strong and keep on the course You've placed before me. Amen.

Reflection

Besides God, who is cheering you on at the finish line?

_____

_____

_____

_____

_____

_____

_____

_____

_____

_____

_____

_____

_____

DAY 37

Rest Stop

And God blessed the seventh day and declared it holy,
because it was the day when he rested from all his work of creation.

—Genesis 2:3

I am a huge multitasker. There. I admit it. I feel I need to constantly be doing something. It's extremely difficult for me to sit and be still. In fact, my husband doesn't believe that those words are even in my vocabulary.

Society tells us keeping busy is how we show we're productive. And since I work from home, my mind believes I need to justify my productivity every day. There seems to be a stigma associated with both working from home and dealing with chronic pain and illness. As a result, I feel that others view me differently.

It's all too easy for me to overdo things. My body tells me when I need to rest or take a break, but my mind doesn't always listen. Unfortunately, when I don't, I regret it, particularly the next day.

God found it important to rest and rejuvenate—in fact, He designated a day for it—the Sabbath. We are created in His image, so why do we fight it? Why is rest or having downtime viewed in a negative light by so many in today's society? It's hard to say no or relinquish control, but it's important to rest our bodies and minds.

We can give ourselves permission to rest when needed. I try to plan my schedule to include a time for this most days of the week. One of my favorite ways to relax is to listen to worship music. It calms my mind, refreshes my soul, and honors God. Take a few moments today to be still. You can pray, listen to uplifting music or a sound machine, take a nap, or just unplug. Find what works best for you. Spend time with your heavenly Father and feel His healing touch.

Lord, thank You for giving me permission to rest and recharge in You
and with You today. Amen.

Reflection

How will you relax today?

_____

_____

_____

_____

_____

_____

_____

_____

_____

_____

_____

_____

_____

_____

DAY 38

Unshakable Faith

I trust in your unfailing love. I will rejoice because you have rescued me.

—Psalm 13:5

You were created to achieve great things. Before you were born, God had plans for you. Sadly, the enemy has plans for you, too, but his are much different. He wants to keep you stuck where you are, and he has many ways of doing that. Perhaps the number one way is to try and destroy your faith. He also loves to make you doubt yourself and your God-given abilities. Odds are good that on the days when your pain is at an all-time high, it may feel like the enemy has the upper hand and is winning. You may think your prayers are going unheard. However, that's not the case.

David wrote today's verse. He went through many trials, and he likely felt that God wasn't always listening to him. In fact, that's how this psalm begins: "O Lord, how long will you forget me? Forever? How long will you look the other way? How long must I struggle with anguish in my soul?" (Psalm 13:1-2).

Yet in verse five, David is glorifying the Lord. He knew that God was still with him and would fulfill His promises. David chose to focus on God instead of his temporary setbacks and struggles.

Circumstances may seem unexpected or designed to rattle you. But nothing is a surprise to God. He is unshakable. And as a Christ-follower, you can tap into the power of unshakable faith. That faith can overcome whatever the enemy may throw at you, including fear, anxiety, pain, failure, or hopelessness. You just need to activate that faith through prayer. What the enemy uses to tear us down, God uses to build us up and grow our faith. Turn to God and trust that He is always at work and will never leave your side.

Lord, I will not let the enemy win today because
my trust and faith are grounded in You. Amen.

Reflection

How can you activate your unshakable faith today?

_____

_____

_____

_____

_____

_____

_____

_____

_____

_____

_____

_____

_____

_____

DAY 39

Stressed or Blessed?

For our present troubles are small and won't last very long.
Yet they produce for us a glory that vastly outweighs them and will last forever!

—2 Corinthians 4:17

When I turned sixteen, my grandparents gave me a used (but new-to-me) car. I was ecstatic. However, that excitement changed when my car died on me while trying to go down the main street in my small town. My car breaking down was an unexpected trouble, and it certainly outweighed my joy.

Ever since I was hit by a car in 1994, my body has been a bit like my first car. That car broke down unexpectedly on occasion, and so does my body. And when that happens, it never feels like a small, insignificant event.

Like me, whatever challenges you're facing likely don't feel light or momentary at the time either. In fact, life may feel like circumstances are piling one on top of the other, with no end in sight.

Paul, who wrote today's verse, faced many challenges, too, including beatings, lashings, and a stoning. So how could he describe his troubles as "light"? He looked at long-term outcomes and all that can result from placing your faith and trust in Jesus. Paul chose not to have tunnel vision. He looked past those moments and saw the blessings beyond. If Paul can shift his perspective like that, we can learn to do the same. In the moment, it's easy to get weighed down by pain and illness. It can feel never ending. Yet by focusing on the larger picture, the view is different. It's important to remember that Jesus is bigger than any disease, crisis, struggle, or pain the enemy may send our way. Things here on earth are momentary compared to the eternal joy lined up for us in Heaven. We can make the choice today to focus on our blessings instead of life's daily stressors.

Lord, I thank You that You are ever faithful, and I will keep my focus on how big You are compared to everything else. Amen.

Reflection

What blessings can you focus on today?

_____

_____

_____

_____

_____

_____

_____

_____

_____

_____

_____

_____

_____

DAY 40

Tie a Knot and Hang On

And this hope will not lead to disappointment. For we know how dearly God loves us because he has given us the Holy Spirit to fill our hears with his love.

—Romans 5:5

Life is messy, and things can go from bad to worse in the blink of an eye. Flare-ups can occur at any moment, even when you're trying your best to do everything right with managing your triggers. When symptoms appear, it's easy to become upset, overwhelmed, stressed, or even depressed. You may feel like giving up or losing hope.

For many, hope typically involves wishing for a favorable outcome. Worldly hope is founded on irrational thinking, and it often leads to frustration and disappointment.

Biblical hope, on the other hand, is different. That hope is based on blessed assurance and trust in Jesus Christ. It is rooted in God's trustworthiness. A Christian's hope is centered on the Word of God and His promises. It is not based on ourselves or other people, so it is not diminished due to our circumstances. There is an assurance that we have a bright future, even if we don't see it in the moment.

In Romans 5:5, Paul tells us that hope doesn't disappoint because our hope is in God alone. It is one of the many benefits of faith. It cannot be changed by one's circumstances. There will still be challenges and suffering. However, those situations provide a chance for us to grow closer to the Father. Our painful moments are an opportunity to rejoice, knowing that God is using them to build perseverance.

Paul reminds us that our hope will be vindicated. We will never regret placing our hope in God's goodness and faithfulness. He will *always* keep His powerful promises, and chronic pain and illness can't negate that. So, when you feel that you are at the end of your rope, tie a knot and hang on! Place your hope firmly in the Lord. He has you, and He will not let you fall.

Lord, thank You for the hope I have through You—
and that I am secure in any and every situation. Amen.

Reflection

What situation are you secure in today?

_____

_____

_____

_____

_____

_____

_____

_____

_____

_____

_____

DAY 41

Are You There, God?

Answer me when I call to you, O God who declares me innocent.
Free me from my troubles. Have mercy on me and hear my prayer.

—Psalm 4:1

Growing up, one of my favorite books was *Are You There, God? It's Me, Margaret* by Judy Bloom. Margaret is a twelve-year-old girl who doesn't attend church or "have religion," but she does have a very real and very special relationship with God. She knows she can talk to Him *anytime* about *anything*.

I love the title of Blume's book, as it's something I've asked on more than one occasion. Logically, I know He hears me. However, I have questioned whether or not He is really *listening* to the words I'm saying. This is especially true when it seems like I'm praying the same prayer over and over again with no response. Though deep down, I know that's not the case.

David may have felt the same way. He wrote Psalm 4:1. And he wasn't just speaking this message for his own benefit. While we don't know David's exact circumstances, we can tell that he was crying out to God, begging to be heard. David's distress is evident. Still, he placed his trust in God, knowing God was listening to each and every word. David was bold in his prayers, asking God to answer him.

Just like with David, God hears your prayers—*all* of them, even the unspoken requests you make when you're in too much pain to string words together. Your prayers may not always be answered in the way you'd like. A response or resolution may not arrive as soon as you'd like. However, it doesn't mean God isn't listening or that He doesn't care. He is not necessarily saying no. Perhaps God is saying, "The time isn't right just yet." God is *always* at work on your behalf. He has a plan for every single event that has happened in your life, even the painful ones. He is lining things up—orchestrating everything down to the tiniest detail. So be like David in today's verse. Go before God. Call out to Him. Pray bold prayers. He's listening.

Lord, help me to be patient, trusting that You have a plan and You will answer my prayers in Your perfect timing. Amen.

Reflection

In what way has God shown you that He hears your prayers?

_____

_____

_____

_____

_____

_____

_____

_____

_____

_____

_____

_____

_____

DAY 42

Above All Else

Yes, everything else is worthless when compared with the infinite value of knowing Christ Jesus my Lord. For his sake I have discarded everything else, counting it all as garbage, so that I could gain Christ and become one with him.

—Philippians 3:8-9

To others, many chronic pain sufferers look the same as anyone else on the outside. They may have a steady job, a loving family, a nice car, and a beautiful house. But what people can't see is all that is going on inside that person and how agonizing it is to maintain a "perfect" front, to attend events in a pain-induced fog, barely going through the motions. To appear "normal" is a daily struggle for many, since society often defines someone by what they can or cannot do.

Chronic pain causes many people to give up on the things they love to do, often in an attempt to just get through the day without having a full-blown flare-up. Changes are made—dreams and plans lost or forgotten—as life unravels one piece at a time.

Paul wrote Philippians 3:8-9. In many ways, he wasn't all that different from us. He is often viewed as a man who lived a good and holy life. That image doesn't make it easy to see him as an example of the average person. The truth is that he, too, was a mere mortal. It took many years for him to become an apostle. He experienced great success and notoriety, but he understood the pain of tremendous loss as well. He grieved and suffered, yet he still valued his relationship with Jesus above everything else. We can follow his example of looking to Jesus and following Him.

Like Paul, it's okay for us to grieve what we've lost. Also like Paul, we can find joy in what can be gained along the way—a deeper, stronger relationship with Jesus. Daily successes are nowhere near as important. While physical healing may not occur this side of Heaven, spiritual healing and strengthening can.

Lord, thank You that through all I've lost due to my illness and pain,
I've gained much more in my relationship with You. Amen.

Reflection

What have you learned about God since your pain journey began?

_____

_____

_____

_____

_____

_____

_____

_____

_____

_____

_____

_____

DAY 43

Through the Fire

My health may fail, and my spirit may grow weak,
but God remains the strength of my heart; he is mine forever.

—Psalm 73:26

It's easy for discouragement and fear to take root when you deal with chronic pain and chronic illness. Life is turned upside down, perhaps on a daily basis. Guilt creeps in when we realize it's impossible to enjoy the event we've been waiting months to attend or offer solace to our crying child. In fact, with our physical and emotional strength zapped, there are times we can barely comfort ourselves.

However, we can look to Psalm 73:26 for encouragement during those difficult times. The verse serves as a reminder that God is always there, and He is our Portion and Strength. Strength can't be purchased or easily replaced through human efforts. Our strength is only replenished as a gift from God, where it shines through our weakness and pain.

We may grow weary and lack confidence while trying to stay afloat with all life throws at us. Feelings of discouragement are normal. But it's important to remember God is taking on our struggles and pain for us.

Today's verse is a reminder that our health may fail, but, thankfully, we do not have to depend on our own human faculties. We have the One Who is strong when we are not. God may bring us to the end of our ropes in order for us to learn to depend on Him and His power, but He will never leave us.

He will be there with us. He is the true Source of our strength. The One Who can help us take that next breath or step when we're convinced it's impossible. The Lord can assist us when we feel we can't take another step. He is the true Source of our provision. He'll give us strength to persevere and endure the perilous journey known as chronic illness.

Lord, thank You for Your strength when I feel too weak
and my journey seems too daunting to navigate alone. Amen.

Reflection

In what area can God give you strength today?

_____

_____

_____

_____

_____

_____

_____

_____

_____

_____

_____

_____

_____

DAY 44

Keep the Faith

And he said to her, "Daughter, your faith has made you well.
Go in peace. Your suffering is over."

—Mark 5:34

"Walk by Faith" is one of my favorite songs by Jeremy Camp. In addition to being a great song, the lyrics are a reminder to release your concerns to the Lord, have faith, trust that He hears you, and allow Him to guide your every step.

Faith is defined as a firm belief in something for which there is no proof, which is sometimes easier said than done. Many days, I wonder why God hasn't healed me or lessened my pain, especially when I have seen others have different results. I would guess you have had similar thoughts. In truth, those questions are something that may not be answered until we get to Heaven. At that time, full healing *will* take place—of that I am confident because the Bible tells us so.

In Mark 5:34, healing came as a result of the woman's faith, which she expressed by touching Jesus's robe. That single act changed her life. She was confident in her faith, in Who Jesus was, and in the fact that He would do what He said He would do. She is the only person in the New Testament to be called "daughter." Jesus claims her as His own and doesn't look down on her, like she anticipates based on how others treat her. Her faith may not have been perfect, but it was focused on the correct person. She sees Jesus; she knows she needs Him; and she is bold enough to follow her faith. That faith is what led to her healing. That same scriptural promise from the Old Testament is as true today as it was then. Like the woman in the verse, we can call out to the Lord and have faith that He claims us as His own. The enemy hates it when we exercise our faith, as it releases God's power. Healing may not occur on our timetable, but we can be confident that, with faith, it *will* happen.

Lord, I have faith that You will keep Your promises
and fill me with Your strength. Amen.

Reflection

What are you clinging to in faith today?

_____

_____

_____

_____

_____

_____

_____

_____

_____

_____

_____

_____

_____

_____

DAY 45

Time-Out

Jesus often withdrew to the wilderness for prayer.

—Luke 5:16

Life can be overwhelming. Deadlines. Finances. Traffic. Children. Illness. On the go. Always connected. We are bombarded from the moment the alarm goes off until we go to bed. And for some people, it doesn't completely stop then. The disruptions continue into the evening and lead to fragmented sleep. Day in and day out, the cycle continues: alarm, work, football game, supper, bills. The stress is compounded when you throw in chronic pain or illness. When do we have a chance to take a breath? Or listen for God's still, small voice?

Luke reminds us that Jesus needed time to step away. After a day of teaching and healing, He took a moment to withdraw from the crowds, find solitude, and spend time talking to His Father—and listening. He was God in the flesh, yet Jesus still needed to pray. He was bombarded with more tasks than we could ever imagine. Sure, He didn't have an overflowing inbox or school events to attend. However, He ministered to thousands of people, and the crowds asking for healing or understanding multiplied daily. As the only Son of God, Jesus was a busy man. Even with all those demands, He knew the importance of having a time-out.

Life pulls us in many directions. On good days, that hectic schedule may be somewhat manageable. But on the not-so-good days? Burnout could occur. If Jesus needed a time to be still, why should we be any different? Why do we feel obligated to be available to everyone at any time of the day? Simply put, if we are too busy to pray, we are too busy. Try something new today. Give yourself permission to turn off the phone and TV. Wait to reply to the emails. Have a moment of silence. Spend some time with your heavenly Father, and see what He wants to tell you today.

Lord, let me hear Your voice today above all the noise around me. Amen.

Reflection

What are you giving yourself permission to set aside today?

_____

_____

_____

_____

_____

_____

_____

_____

_____

_____

_____

_____

_____

DAY 46

Our Cheerleader

What shall we say about such wonderful things as these?
If God is for us, who can ever be against us?

—Romans 8:31

If, like me, you are dealing with chronic pain or chronic illness, you know how frustrating it is when you are unable to do what you used to do, want to do, or enjoy doing. Your body is saying it's just too much, so you need to alter your plans. Shopping or laundry may have to wait. It can feel like everyone and everything (including your own body) is against you.

The enemy may try to make you believe that God is working against you. Some people envision God sitting with a checklist, marking down everything they've done wrong so He can dole out punishment. You may have been led to believe that your chronic pain and illness is a result of that. However, that isn't how God operates. He loves you. He is working in everything for your good. He is on your side—always.

In Romans 8:31, Paul tells us that God is for us. He is on our side, and that's all we truly need to know. Nothing can change that, not even pain or illness. After all, He gave up His Son so that we can always be with Him.

Faith isn't about removing our pain or the trials we face. Paul could attest to that fact. He knew we'd be tested. If Paul were here today, he would remind you that Jesus conquered it all. It may feel at times that you're swimming upstream against the current. Don't fear. You can rest assured that God will bring healing and deliverance, in His time, according to His will and plans. He is on your side. And with Him there, no one can ever be against you. So put your trust in Him and rely on His love. He's rooting for you!

Lord, thank You for loving me, encouraging me, supporting me,
and always being in my corner. Amen.

Reflection

How has God reminded you that He is on your side, cheering you on?

_____

_____

_____

_____

_____

_____

_____

_____

_____

_____

_____

_____

_____

DAY 47

Wonderfully Made

*You made all the delicate, inner parts of my body and knit me together in my
mother's womb. Thank you for making me so wonderfully complex!
Your workmanship is marvelous—how well I know it.*

—Psalm 139:13-14

Before my feet even hit the floor in the morning, the muscle pain spreads throughout my body. Staying in bed isn't even an option, based on the shooting pains in my hip and shoulder. And with each tiny movement and breath, I can tell that my plans for the day will need adjusting. I try to block out the negative voices in my head telling me I'm useless and that I should just give up. I can't help but wish I could wake up in someone else's body, one without aches and pains—if only for one day.

On days like this, it's hard to believe that I'm "wonderfully made." Yet that's exactly what I am, and the same is true for you, too. No one is perfect.

Our pain and illness are not a surprise to God. Wishing we were different or someone else is pointless. We are exactly as we are meant to be, precisely as God made us to be. It may be hard to see in the moment, but God made us uniquely complex for a purpose no one else can fulfill. We are still works in progress and part of God's grand design.

Everyone has something they would like to change about themselves. But when we learn to view ourselves through God's eyes, our perspective shifts. God accepted us into His family, and it came at a high cost—the life of His

Son, the precious blood of Jesus. Genesis 1:27 states that we are all created in the image of God. He breathed life into us, and He is pleased with us *just as we are.* God doesn't look at you and see your imperfections. He sees you as His daughter, one who is "fearfully and wonderfully made." Nothing about you is a mistake. Do not allow pain or the enemy to deceive you into thinking anything different. You are precious and valuable.

Lord, I choose to praise You for the wonderful way You created me,
knowing that even my pain and weaknesses are valuable and useful to You. Amen.

Reflection

What negative voices are you blocking out today and replacing with God's truths?

_____

_____

_____

_____

_____

_____

_____

_____

_____

_____

_____

_____

_____

DAY 48

Give to Receive

Give, and you will receive. Your gift will return to you in full—pressed down, shaken together to make room for more, running over, and poured into your lap. The amount you give will determine the amount you get back.

—Luke 6:38

I recently had the opportunity to help a friend in need in the simplest way. She needed someone to be there—even though it was over the phone—for her to talk with as she created a memorial wreath for her brother. I was honored to be the person who could help her out in her time of need.

By helping her, I also helped myself. I'd been in a flare-up all day. Did my migraine, tingling sensations, and spasms suddenly disappear? No, but for a short time, I was able to take my mind off my own painful situation and shift my focus to my friend's needs. She was grateful that I took time out of my day to spend a few moments with her. I was equally thankful to her for allowing me to be there when she needed someone. Days later, I told her how much it meant to me to have had that time with her. My friend was surprised to learn that she had helped me as much, if not more, than I'd helped her.

Luke 6:38 is often applied to money, but it truly references so much more, including compassion, mercy, forgiveness, understanding, and patience. Yet it's also a reminder that we reap what we sow. As I witnessed in helping my friend, when blessings go from person to person, they also come down from God to us.

God blesses us, so we can bless others in whatever way is possible at any given time. My friend needed someone to listen as she completed a love-filled task at a difficult time. I needed some task to distract me and interrupt my pain cycle. I was glad I could be there for her—giving freely, expecting nothing in return. Take a moment to look around—outside yourself—to see if you can be there for someone else today.

Lord, I want to use the gifts and resources You've given me
to bless others and bring glory to Your name. Amen.

Reflection

Who can you bless today?

_____

_____

_____

_____

_____

_____

_____

_____

_____

_____

_____

DAY 49

Facing the Giants

"The Lord who rescued me from the claws of the lion and the bear will rescue me from this Philistine!" Saul finally consented. "All right, go ahead," he said. "And may the LORD be with you!"

—1 Samuel 17:37

Living with a chronic illness can be scary, particularly when new symptoms arise. For some, those moments result in a trip to the emergency room, where a long wait to be seen increases fears and anxieties. Each new symptom and diagnosis feels like another mountain to climb.

Everyone faces a giant of one kind or another at some point in life. That didn't just start with the modern generation. Today's verse is a reminder of that. Samuel tells us that David feared, but God rescued him. The Lord was with David, and He is with us as well.

David had spent his life as a shepherd. He faced lions and bears while protecting his sheep. He never realized he was training to fight a giant named Goliath. David knew God delivered him in the past, so he was sure that would be the case again. God's strength allowed David to defeat Goliath, an achievement few would have thought likely. And it would have been impossible without God by David's side. Like David, God is preparing us as well, even if we're not sure about the specific details. Pain can cloud our memories. It may also block out reminders of when God provided for us and delivered us from numerous giants of our own or allowed us to take part in events we thought would be impossible for fear of a flare-up. With a chronic illness, our bodies are the perfect environment for what-if thoughts that lock us in a prison of fears. Second Timothy 1:7 is a reminder that God did not give us a spirit of fear.

Look to the Lord to hold you up when facing new symptoms. Turn to the Lord, not the internet. Instead of being held captive, allow Him to rescue you from the swirling thoughts and anxieties.

Lord, thank You for the reminders of how You've been there for me in the past and that I can run to You instead of fearing the giants I may face. Amen.

Reflection

When has God helped you defeat giants in the past?

_____

_____

_____

_____

_____

_____

_____

_____

_____

_____

_____

DAY 50

I Will Trust in You

But when I am afraid, I will put my trust in you.

—Psalm 56:3

I don't know about you, but I had big aspirations as a child. I wanted to write, teach, sing, and travel around the world—but maybe not all of them at the same time. However, chronic pain and illness were never a part of those plans. Yet years later, that's now my life. It may be yours, too.

Sometimes, it takes all I have to not run to "Dr. Google" and check to see if my new symptom is something to be concerned about or if it is just another one to add to the growing list. And of course, when I do give in and look things up, the symptoms are almost always something serious, which fires up my anxiety and causes ten thousand thoughts—mostly fears—to run through my mind.

David knew what fear was, and he had plenty of reasons to be afraid. In fact, he didn't say *"if* I am afraid" but *"when* I am afraid." Unlike David, most of us don't have his concerns of fleeing from his son, Absalom, who pursued David with the intent to kill him and take over the throne. However, in addition to those fears, David knew something else—placing your trust in God will transform fear into faith. You can't handle everything on your own—but God can (1 Peter 5:7).

The Bible tells us, "Don't be afraid" (Isa. 41:10), and the best way to do that is to bombard fear with faith. The enemy targets our fears. He amplifies them and preys on them. He uses them to increase our insecurity, anxiety, and distress. *Faith,* however, will attack the fear that tries to blind us to the reality that God is in control. He never leaves us. He is the ultimate Physician. And most importantly, He loves us unconditionally.

Lord, I will trust in You instead of being overwhelmed by my irrational fears. Amen.

Reflection

What fears will you trust God with today?

_____

_____

_____

_____

_____

_____

_____

_____

_____

_____

_____

_____

_____

_____

DAY 51

Our Comforter

All praise to God, the Father of our Lord Jesus Christ. God is our merciful Father and the source of all comfort. He comforts us in all our troubles so that we can comfort others. When they are troubled, we will be able to give them the same comfort God has given us.

—2 Corinthians 1:3-4

I remember crawling up into my gram's lap when I was small. Whether I was scared, sick, or tired, she seemed to make it all better with a hug, a smile, and a few comforting words. Have you ever wanted to do that as an adult? There are many forms of comfort in our modern world—from food and water to shelter or entertainment. However, crawling up into someone's lap to make everything feel better might not be as effective or practical for an adult as it is for a child. Our grown-up minds are more logical. We know that problems don't just magically disappear with a caring touch or words of comfort. Or do they? We are never too old to benefit from someone comforting us, encouraging us, giving us strength, or revitalizing our hope.

Paul wrote today's verse, and he understood the need for that same comfort, encouragement, and strength. He was often overwhelmed and faced with situations beyond his human abilities. He was imprisoned, beaten, and faced death time and time again. He knew pain. Nevertheless, Paul also knew where to turn.

The Greek word for comfort is *άνεση*, and it's defined as "to give strength and hope" or "to ease the grief or trouble of." God is the ultimate Father, and He has given us the Holy Spirit to minister to and empower us. Paul was all too familiar with this concept as he reminds us in 2 Corinthians 1:3. God invites us to come to Him—any time, any place, for any reason. His encouragement inspires hope, and His compassion is always available. He will help us endure whatever may come our way.

Lord, thank You for knowing my heart, caring about my concerns,
and offering comfort when I'm in need. Amen.

Reflection

How will you find solace in God today?

_____

_____

_____

_____

_____

_____

_____

_____

_____

_____

_____

DAY 52

You Are Enough

Should the thing that was created say to the one who created it,
"Why have you made me like this?"

—Romans 9:20

In today's society, it is easy to focus on what you have or don't have or to find fault with various things in your life. There is a temptation to compare yourself to others and wonder if you're good enough, smart enough, talented enough, pretty enough, healthy enough, productive enough, or successful enough. It's human nature to ask these questions on occasion.

However, have you ever stopped to think of the fact that God made you *exactly* as He wanted you to be? If you were meant to be taller, you would be taller. If you were supposed to look a certain way, you would. And if you were meant to be free from chronic pain and illness, God would have done that, too. He is the Master Potter. He knows what He's doing, even if we don't.

There is no point in focusing on the what-if questions. Everyone is flawed, but flawed doesn't mean ruined. God doesn't owe us an explanation on anything. Everyone has something they'd like to change about themselves. So, you're not alone in wondering, "Why me?" A better question to ask is, "Why *not* me?" Christ-followers are not promised a trouble-free or pain-free life.

God has a purpose for *you* that no one can fulfill *except you*. He is constantly shaping you. Every part of you—including your chronic pain and illness—is the way it is for a purpose, so don't resist who you are. If you're struggling today, ask God for help. Ask Him to show you how He sees you. Trust Him. Stop comparing yourself to others. You were made for a specific purpose, so go out there and be the best you that you can be. No one else can do it for you. Honor God with your uniqueness.

Lord, thank You that I'm uniquely made and that You love me for me. Amen.

Reflection

What is one way that you're unique?

_____

_____

_____

_____

_____

_____

_____

_____

_____

_____

_____

_____

_____

DAY 53

A Balanced Life

"Be still and know that I am God!"

—Psalm 46:10

I don't know about you, but I multitask on a regular basis. It's hard for me not to when there are so many things I want to accomplish each day. And if I've recently had a bad day with a flare-up that prevented me from completing my to-do list, the list of things I need or want to achieve is even longer.

It's always been difficult for me to be still. I have problems relaxing. I think, in part, it's because I don't want to allow my mind the downtime to kick into overdrive and run away with my fears, anxieties, and what-if thoughts. I also worry that my chronic illness will cause others to view me as lazy or weak. However, by not allowing myself the time to just be, I not only shut those thoughts out, but I also shut out God's voice, which is *not* my intent at all. The challenge is to find the balance where I can be still enough to hear God, yet also block out the negativity fighting for a prime-time spot in my mind and life. It's definitely a work in progress, and it may be for you, too.

In today's society, it's hard to slow down our bodies *and* minds. It goes against our nature and culture, which encourage us to charge ahead at full speed. Psalm 46:10 is a popular verse for many to memorize, for good reason. It's a reminder that it's okay to stop striving so hard. You don't need to prove yourself to anyone. God longs to talk to us, but He will never force us to listen. We should *want* to listen. It's an honor to do so. It's a privilege to be a child of God. Set aside time today to take a few deep breaths. Close your eyes. Be still. Listen to what your Father wants to tell you.

Lord, quiet my mind and allow me to feel Your peace and stillness today. Amen.

Reflection

What can you do today to allow yourself to hear what God is saying to you?

_____

_____

_____

_____

_____

_____

_____

_____

_____

_____

_____

_____

_____

_____

_____

_____

DAY 54

Simple Truths

"Do not be afraid or discouraged, for the Lord will personally go ahead of you.
He will be with you; he will neither fail you nor abandon you."

—Deuteronomy 31:8

Chronic pain and chronic illness are such solitary things to live with. You *look* perfectly fine on the outside. Therefore, you *must* be fine, correct? Well, if you are the one experiencing it, you know that statement couldn't be further from the truth.

Chronic illness is complex. Our bodies feel defective or inferior, and there's little we can do about any of it. It's normal to question God. People who don't have a chronic condition often don't get it, so it's easy to feel isolated. However, that's not true either. You aren't alone. Here are some simple truths to remember today:

- *God sees you.* He is there in the gentle breeze you feel on your face and in every breath you take. No matter the situation, God is there (Josh. 1:9).
- *God is with you.* He is beside you, behind you, and in front of you always (Psalm 139:5).
- *God knows you.* He created you in His image, and He knows you better than anyone. He has counted the number of hairs on your head. He's called you by name, and you are His child (Isa. 43:1).

- *God loves you.* God never promised a pain-free life, but He did promise to be with you and get you through it (Deut. 31:8).
- *You are not your illness or pain.* That is just one part of you, but it doesn't need to define you (2 Cor. 5:17).

During a flare-up, the enemy may try to convince you that you're alone and that God has abandoned you. The enemy wants you to give in, to quit, and to focus on the negatives. Remind the enemy that Christ is by your side. With Him, there is nothing you can't do. He will be your strength when you feel weak (Phil. 4:13). Go back and reread today's verse. Memorize it. Find solace in it. And take comfort in the Lord.

Lord, thank You for Your faithfulness to walk beside me today,
no matter the circumstance. Amen.

Reflection

Which of God's truths do you need to cling to today?

_____

_____

_____

_____

_____

_____

_____

_____

_____

_____

DAY 55

System Overload

The Lord is my shepherd; I have all that I need.
He lets me rest in green meadows; he leads me beside peaceful streams.

—Psalm 23:1-2

Our bodies know when we need rest. Logically, I know that. However, I'm not always good at listening to what my body is telling me. I tend to push my limits. A specialist put things in perspective for me at a recent visit. He explained that our bodies are like a fuse box. My increased symptoms were due to system overload. As a result, my "fuses" are now acting out and firing at random. This was not the news I wanted to hear. It's challenging enough to handle the symptoms, which are somewhat predictable. Now I'm told that they'll be more unexpected? It was a bit hard to feel positive after that appointment.

Thankfully, the Lord blessed me with a flexible career. That's beneficial for the fluctuations in my symptoms. I'm able to work at a slower pace and take breaks when needed. As David mentions in Psalm 23:1-2, it's important to have that time to rest when my body tells me I need to do so—even if, on occasion, I require a reminder.

Since that doctor visit, I've gotten (a bit) better at taking time to relax and recharge on a more regular basis. In fact, there have been times that I've actually written it in my calendar as a scheduled appointment with the Lord.

Over time, I've come to see the blessing in these moments. They allow me to spend time with my Father. I'm thankful for these moments of rest. My body thanks me for it. Yours will as well. Give it a try. Listen to what your body is telling you. Allow yourself to have a few minutes of downtime. David knew that sheep trust their shepherd, and we can trust ours, too. The Lord will give us peace and rest if we allow Him to do so.

Lord, help me to realize that it's okay to quiet my mind and spirit and savor those moments where I slow down and spend time with You. Amen.

Reflection

How can you add more rest time into your daily schedule?

_____

_____

_____

_____

_____

_____

_____

_____

_____

_____

_____

_____

_____

DAY 56

Infinite Value

But God showed his great love for us by sending Christ
to die for us while we were still sinners.

—Romans 5:8

Our pastor once pulled out a crisp fifty-dollar bill during his sermon. He asked if anyone wanted it. Hands went up all over the auditorium. Of course, many people were interested in the money. The pastor then did various things to the bill, such as writing on it, crumbling it into a ball, dropping it on the floor, then stomping on it. He once again asked if anyone wanted the money. Many hands still went up. He asked why anyone would want it, as it's now damaged. Someone near the back of the room yelled out, "Yeah, but it's still worth fifty dollars!"

Our pastor handed the money to that person, then went on with his message—a crumpled fifty-dollar bill is still valuable, and so are crumpled, damaged, or hurting people. God still views us as crisp, clean, and worthy. So much so, in fact, that He sent His son to die for us—with our bruises, sins, illnesses, and imperfections.

Even when we feel like we're a mess, God still wants us. He still loves us. In fact, His amazing love is not dependent on us being deserving. He loved us before we even knew Him. He gave His Son for us. We don't need to be cleaned up or perfected. God's love is based on the fact that God is love, and He extends that love to everyone. We can go to Him with the good, the bad, and the ugly. In spite of our shortcomings, we are precious to Him. He longs to have a relationship with us, just as we are. He wants us to reach out to Him, to turn to Him, to trust Him, and to love Him. His love is unconditional. Chronic pain and illness can never change that fact.

Lord, thank You that even when I don't feel worthy, perfect, or put together,
I am still valuable to You. Amen.

Reflection

How did God demonstrate His love for you today?

_____

_____

_____

_____

_____

_____

_____

_____

_____

_____

_____

_____

_____

_____

DAY 57

Perfectly Imperfect

*Each time he said, "My grace is all you need. My power works best in weakness."
So now I am glad to boast about my weaknesses, so that the power of Christ
can work through me.*

—2 Corinthians 12:9

I'm a list-maker, big time! I can't tell you the last time I did something spontaneous. I like to have a schedule to follow for everything, even when traveling or on vacation. I expect perfection from myself (and often others). It's no surprise, I'm sure, that this rarely happens. It's also no surprise that my way of thinking often leads to increased stress and pain.

My husband is the opposite. It's far easier for him to go with the flow. He's constantly telling me to "breathe," "relax," or "let it go." On many occasions, he's helped me see the bright side of things or admit that the world is still turning, even if my plans for the day were totally flipped on their head.

I've tried to imitate his easygoing attitude, and it works for me—sometimes. In fact, my phrase one year was "Shake it off." I admit that I often failed. One day when my pain and stress levels were through the roof, I took my blood pressure. It was much higher than it's ever been. *That* was a wake-up call for me.

Perfection is even more difficult to find when dealing with chronic pain and illness. Society tells us to "get over it" or "just deal with it and move on." Many of us are wired to be on alert and striving for the best at all times. How much aggravation do I—and perhaps you—cause by expecting perfection from an imperfect body? A feat that is only accomplished by Jesus. It's challenging, but I'm learning to have patience with myself and remember that God uses those weaknesses I try to gloss over. He still loves me as I am— perfectly imperfect.

Lord, when I struggle for perfection, remind me that it's okay to be human and that You love me, flaws and all. Amen.

Reflection

What phrase or word can remind you to go easier on yourself?

_____

_____

_____

_____

_____

_____

_____

_____

_____

_____

_____

_____

_____

_____

_____

DAY 58

Daily Strength

Search for the LORD and for his strength; continually seek him.

—Psalm 105:4

Life is hard for everyone. For someone dealing with chronic pain or illness, that statement is even more accurate, especially when others are unable to see or feel what's going on inside of your body and mind. There are days when it's a struggle to do the most basic things, such as climb out of bed, shower, get dressed, or make a meal.

I have a daily routine that I try to follow, even when I'm traveling. I begin each day in prayer, even before I get out of bed. I lie there for a few moments in silence. It's the perfect time to ask God for strength to do His will that day and to listen for what He wants to tell me.

Listening may not always be easy throughout the course of the day when life threatens to overwhelm you with all there is to do. But as David reminds us in Psalm 105:4, it's important to seek God and His strength. That's why I try to read my Bible and do my devotions before breakfast, so I'm sure to get the time in before the daily tasks take over. Some days, I don't accomplish as much as I'd like to do, and it's frustrating. However, the day was still a success because I spent time with God, which is the most important task I can do. And it's the most important thing you can do, too.

Take a few minutes today to get quiet before God and see what He has to say to you. He will be as close as you allow Him to be. He will give you the strength you need. Watch for His presence in your daily life. I assure you, He's right there with you.

Lord, when I feel weak, I will turn to You because with You, I am strong. Amen.

Reflection

What did God say to you today during your quiet time?

_____

_____

_____

_____

_____

_____

_____

_____

_____

_____

_____

_____

_____

_____

_____

_____

DAY 59

Unburdened

The Sovereign LORD is my strength!

—Habakkuk 3:19

There are many times I've wanted to give up or not make a change. I've been afraid that I couldn't do a task or activity because of my pain and illness. I've learned that sometimes, it's easier to suffer in silence. Sure, I may miss out on something, but I won't end up burdening anyone else. Deep down, I know my family and friends don't view me that way. However, it's not always easy to remember that in the moment, when the enemy throws his barbs my way.

If you've ever felt that you're a burden, take a look at what Romans 8:28 has to say: "And we know that God causes everything to work together for the good of those who love God." That verse tells us that God is working *everything* for our good.

On more than one occasion, God has given me strength to get through a situation or complete so many things I didn't think possible—from being strong for my husband during his surgery to becoming a published author. Both were things I never would have imagined a few years ago. Yet God had different plans.

At the beginning of Habakkuk, the prophet questions God. In verse 3:18, Habakkuk rejoiced in his trials. Then in 3:19, he recognizes where his strength comes from. Habakkuk didn't understand God's ways or timing. We may not understand either. However, that doesn't mean we have to doubt His love or question His wisdom. It's possible to stand firm in God, even when it feels like the world around us is crumbling. Habakkuk went from questions to doubt to confusion to faith, then on to hope and confidence. He learned to trust. We can also learn to have that same confidence in God, even in the midst of chaos or the unknowns associated with chronic pain and illness.

Lord, help me trust in You even when my world is turned upside down. Amen.

Reflection

When has God given you strength to get through a difficult situation?

_____

_____

_____

_____

_____

_____

_____

_____

_____

_____

_____

_____

_____

_____

DAY 60

Don't Settle

For God is working in you, giving you the desire and the power to do what pleases him.

—Philippians 2:13

I read something online that caused me to pause. It was a post about how we should upgrade our beliefs to match our visions versus giving up on dreams that may not match our current reality. This was something I'd never considered before, but it made me realize that that was exactly what I'd done. I had downgraded my dreams over the past two decades since my battle with chronic pain and illness began. I had stopped believing I could have a productive, happy life.

As a child and teen, I had grand plans. Like many people, I didn't think anything could stop me from being what I wanted to be and doing everything I wanted to do. My way of thinking changed after my initial diagnosis in 1994. Looking back, I can see how that event led me to expect nothing more than a mediocre life at best, due to my new normal. Thankfully, God had other plans. He reminded me that He wasn't through with me yet.

That social media post was the wake-up call I needed to change my perspective. Chronic pain and illness does *not* have to steal my hope, joy, or dreams. It doesn't have to steal yours either.

Each of us was created for a specific purpose. As long as we're here on earth, God is still using us. He has plans for us. We can trust Him and honor

Him with our thoughts, words, and actions. While *your plans* may have changed as a result of chronic pain and illness, *His calling* on your life has not. As God's children, we have no reason to settle for anything less than God's best for our lives. Years of struggling with chronic pain and illness can take a toll on a person's mind, body, and spirit. However, God is the Source of all hope. It's never too late to begin expecting His goodness in your life. You are valuable and precious to Him. There's no need to settle for anything less.

Lord, don't allow me to settle for anything less than what
You have lined up for me. Amen.

Reflection

Where have you been settling lately?

APPENDIX A

Advice for the Newly Diagnosed

There are so many things I know now that I wish I had known years ago when I was first diagnosed with a chronic illness. At that time, I had no idea how much it would change every area of my life. I was clueless about the emotional roller coaster ride that accompanies such a diagnosis. And that search for a diagnosis can take time as well—sometimes years. (For me, it took ten years.) Many people have coexisting conditions, which can make finding that diagnosis even more of a challenge. Having that "name" won't make things automatically better, but it is reassuring to have confirmation that it's not all in your mind.

After I received my diagnosis, I expected I'd recover. I didn't fully grasp the toll a chronic illness would take on me physically and emotionally. I had studied psychology in college, so I had a basic idea of the stages a person experiences when dealing with grief—denial, anger, bargaining, depression, and acceptance. But no one told me that I'd go through those same stages of grief after receiving my diagnosis. Initially, I found it hard to believe that I'd grieve, as I was still alive and hadn't lost anyone. However, my grief (and yours, too) is for the life I *thought* I'd have, where the future seemed wide open; the life I *did* have, where I could do just about whatever I wanted to do whenever I wanted to do it; and the life I no longer have, where I now need to make adjustments and rest on a regular basis. You can't properly grieve until you've gone through the cycle, which includes denial, fear, and worry. It's a process that will take time, and it may be something that comes and goes as the pain and illness wax and wane.

The provider who gave me my diagnosis never explained any of this to me. And that's why I want to give you a bit of information I wish I'd received years ago.

1. *It's okay to grieve.* It's important to remember that you can still live a happy life and accomplish your dreams. Things just may not unfold in the manner and timeframe you originally envisioned. You're allowed to experience a wide range of emotions, the same as anyone else, including those without a chronic illness. Sadness and crying are not signs of weakness. They are signs that you're human.

2. *Be gentle and patient with yourself.* It will take some time, but you will eventually find a new normal. It's important to keep an open mind. Be willing to make changes and try new things. Take a deep breath, and approach things one day (and one step) at a time. Don't be afraid to ask for help when needed. You will have good days and bad days. You may need to take regular breaks or rest more often than others. And that is perfectly fine. Never feel guilty for doing what you need to do to take care of yourself. Set small, perhaps daily, goals and focus on those. Don't get stuck on what you didn't get done. Concentrate on what you *did* do. There are some parts of your illness that cannot be changed, no matter what you do or don't do. Search for the wisdom to know the difference and make the changes you can make. And be patient and accepting of those things you cannot change.

Having a sense of humor is also important. I have word-finding issues on occasion, thanks to "fibro fog." It's frustrating, for sure, but there's little I can do about it but accept it for what it is. My husband has helped me find the humor in the times when

I call the can opener our "other toaster" or refer to Big Lots as "the other Best Buy."

3. *Find a support system.* It's important to have our loved ones around us, but it's also beneficial to find others going through a similar experience. They will have an in-depth understanding that your loved ones may not have. That connection is why I created my Hope Amid the Pain Facebook group (www.facebook. com/groups/hopeamidthepain) and Instagram page (www. instagram.com/hopeamidthepain). To find a support system that works for you, you may need to reach out to strangers, online and/or in person. When you find your tribe, navigating a life of chronic pain and illness will be a bit easier and smoother. You'll be able to connect with those who have been there, done that. In my experience, these people are more than willing to give advice on what worked for them and what they've learned over the course of their journeys. There are also a number of national organizations specific to your particular diagnosis that will be helpful and informative. A list of some places you can find support are listed in the resources section of this book.

Find what works best for you. Do your research. Seek out others who are knowledgeable about your condition. Learn what you can. Then tweak things and apply them to your daily life and living situation. Don't let others decide for you. Choose what you can implement and what works best for you. Everything won't fall into place immediately. This will involve a lot of trial and error. Chronic illness can affect every area in your life, and you may need to make numerous changes—to goals, relationships, and even daily routines. Life throws curveballs at everyone, but you are strong enough to handle it. There's not one answer that will work for everyone. You may have to adjust your wardrobe to include fewer buttons or zippers. You may need to request easy-open prescription bottles from your pharmacy. Online delivery versus in-person shopping may be less draining. With patience and practice, you'll find a new normal that works best for you and your lifestyle.

4. *Advocate for yourself.* This one is huge! *No one* knows your body like you do. Doctors are knowledgeable, but they don't know everything about every illness. And they don't know you. Doctors are busy, and they see a lot of patients. You need to be prepared when you go to your appointments. Write down your questions in advance. Take a notebook and pen with you or another person, so you remember what is discussed. Be sure to express what is going on—your questions and concerns—as best you can and as precisely as possible. A medical professional will only be as helpful as the information they receive from you. Many other people may have the same diagnosis as you have, but no one else will experience it in exactly the same way. *You are the expert on you.*

APPENDIX B

Tips and Helpful Hacks

My journey with chronic pain and illness has been a long one (over twenty-five years as of this writing). I've learned that I need to listen to God as well as my body. In general, my mind may be willing to do something, but my body isn't always able to do so.

Knowing that I can rely on God for everything and anything is *huge*! I've seen time and time again confirmation that He is listening to me. He hears my cries and praises. Little reminders of that fact pop up for me on a regular basis. He meets me where I am, and He'll do the same for you.

Over the years, I've learned to adapt a bit. I admit I still find it frustrating that I'm not always able to do what I want to do when I want to do it. Thankfully, I'm blessed with a supportive husband, as well as a career I love that allows me to have flexibility on a daily basis.

Finding what works for you, in many areas, is key, and it will likely only be accomplished through trial and error. I have discovered that regular chiropractor adjustments and massage appointments are beneficial for me. They keep me functioning at the best level possible for me and my diagnoses. I've also found the following things, in no particular order, to be helpful. Perhaps some of them will work for you, too.

- *Spend time with God daily.* This tip is an important one for anyone, even those without chronic pain and illness. I find that setting aside time first thing in the morning to read my Bible and devotionals, as well as journal on what I've read, helps me feel prepared for the day ahead. It also gives me time to listen for what God may want to tell me.

- *Listen to your body and know when to ask for help.* These two go together. They were challenging for me to learn, and they're still a work of progress. My body reminds me that I can't do everything on my own. This includes keeping things around my house that I use on a regular basis at a level that I can easily reach. My husband is tall and helpful, but he is not always around when I need something. I have to be able to get items with minimal stretching, crouching, etc. So, prioritizing what goes on which shelves is one more adjustment I've made. I've also found a grabber tool to be an extremely useful tool to help around the house when my husband isn't around.

- *Play and sing worship music.* Aside from my devotional time, I find that worship music is another way I feel closest to the Lord. Just in general, singing is one of the best stress-reducers you can find. It relaxes the body and mind. So, sing like no one but God is listening to you!

- *Apply ice and heat.* I use both, depending on my pain level and the location. I generally use at least one of them on a daily basis. Some people prefer one over the other, and some pain and causes of pain respond better to one over the other. You may want to discuss your particular situation with your doctor to see which may be best for you and your individual pain.

- *Commit to gentle exercise (as tolerated).* Exercise can be beneficial to everyone, even those with a chronic illness. The level of intensity varies, however, for each person. My tolerance level fluctuates. There are a variety of activities I participate in on an alternating basis. Finding what you enjoy and what works for you is key. Some of the things I like are walking, riding a recumbent bike, yoga, and gentle dancing (such as Zumba Gold, which is designed for those with a chronic illness or older adults). Many options can be found for free on sites such as YouTube. Depending on where you live, there could be in-person options, too. It is a good idea to consult with your doctor before beginning any exercise regimen.

- *Take frequent breaks.* I have a to-do list that I work off of every day, or at least I try to. I've had many people (including doctors, therapists, and loved ones) tell me that I need to take regular breaks. I prefer to work until I get to a good stopping point, but that's not always what my body wants or requires. A couple years ago, I purchased an old-school sand timer. I used to use an electronic timer or one on my phone, but I found that it was too easy for me to ignore them when they went off. The sand timer sits on my desk beside my computer. I can easily see it while working. The timer (which is my favorite color—purple!) serves as a reminder to take regular breaks. And of course, I listen to my body, which may require even more frequent breaks than my thirty-minute timer suggests.

- *Join a support group.* I have found a number of great, supportive groups on Facebook. Online, I have met people who are able to attend in-person groups. I wish that were possible in my area, but it's not. However, it is something you may want to investigate for your locale. While no one in these groups will be able to offer a quick fix or cure, I've found it helpful to know that I'm not alone in what I'm going through.

Again, these are just suggestions. They work for me. They may not be as helpful for you. It will take trial and error to discover what helps you adapt and live your best life. With practice, you will find tips and hacks that are beneficial for you.

APPENDIX C

Creating and Using a Gratitude Journal

Gratitude is often defined as being thankful. It can be the act of showing appreciation for something, as well as returning that kindness. Learning to express gratitude on a regular basis is where a journal comes in and can be helpful. Gratitude journaling can change your life and allow you to reap a number of positive benefits.

Living with chronic pain and illness is challenging. It's sometimes hard to look beyond the moment, especially when you're dealing with the accompanying pain, anxiety, grief, and possibly anger.

A gratitude journal is a tool that can help you shift your focus from something negative to something positive. Journaling is a way to find the good in each situation. It allows you to keep track of the blessings in life that might be masked by pain and flare-ups. By writing and being grateful on a regular basis, you may, over time, discover that you are strengthened and better able to deal with the difficult times when they arise.

Joy is everywhere. But it can easily be overshadowed by pain, if you allow it to do so. For some people, it will take a deliberate effort and regular practice to learn to look for the positives in daily life.

You may wonder how a gratitude journal differs from a diary, planner, or regular notebook. The difference is found in the focus of each.

- A gratitude journal focuses on what you are grateful for. It's centered on noticing the positive things in life.

- A diary focuses on everything, positive or negative, that occurred during your day.
- A planner focuses on the tasks you want or need to do in a day. While it may include events or activities you may or may not want to do, it's generally neutral.
- A notebook is used to take notes on something or to help you remember key points.

So as you can see, there are some similarities. However, each item serves a specific purpose, and they aren't used interchangeably.

Gratitude journaling, and even the journal itself, will be a little different for everyone. There is no one right way. You have to find a schedule and practice what works for you, your routine, and your lifestyle. However, there are some basics to keep in mind that will help you start a gratitude journal, as well as make it a habit you will stick to.

1. *Choose a journal.* The first step in your gratitude journal practice is choosing a journal. Consider which option will work best for you. Some questions to ask yourself are:
   - Do you want a physical journal, or would you prefer to use a digital format?
   - Will you want something you can carry with you, or will you designate a place and time to journal at home?
   - Do you want a lined or unlined notebook? Will you want the option to doodle in the journal, too?

   Standard notebooks are a popular option for many people, as they offer a lot of flexibility. They come in a variety of shapes and sizes, which makes them a portable, durable option. You should choose something that will be used exclusively for journaling. Pick a notebook that inspires you to make gratitude journaling a regular practice. If you're crafty or creative, you may prefer to go with something basic so you can personalize it even further by adding illustrations or pictures of people, places, and things you love.

2. *Focus on the benefits.* It's important to think about the reason for why you do an activity, and that is also true for journaling. If you understand the *why*, you're more likely to stick with it and make it a habit. For instance, many people don't like to exercise or do chores, but, logically, they see the benefits behind doing so. The same is true of gratitude journaling, but you may find it much more enjoyable than exercise or chores!

When battling a chronic illness, painful situations arise on a regular basis. There's not always an obvious trigger, so it may seem unlikely that something so easy as journaling and positive thinking could make a difference. However, the simple act of practicing gratitude on a regular basis truly can bring hope and joy to even the darkest of times. It won't automatically make everything better. However, there are a number of benefits that tend to occur after establishing a journaling routine.

Through writing, you may notice that you feel less stressed, and you may start to view things from a different perspective. Journaling can help you focus on what and who is important to you. It's possible that you may discover a greater appreciation for the "little things" in your daily life. You may even notice blessings in disguise.

On the challenging days when your pain is increased, your journal could serve another benefit. By looking through it and reading what you've written in the past, you will be able to see the good things that have happened in your life. You'll feel more accomplished when you realize your list of achievements, no matter how small they may have seemed at the time. You may notice ways that God has worked in your life and through your struggles. And unlike many treatment options, there are no side effects or noticeable downsides to utilizing a gratitude journal!

3. *Schedule time for writing.* It's not always easy to find time to add one more task to an ever-growing to-do list, especially on days when you're having a flare-up. But by making gratitude journaling a regular part of your schedule, you may soon discover that it actually helps reduce your stress and possibly even your pain level.

Establishing a regular time is key. When you are new to journaling, the thought of writing daily may be overwhelming. If that's the case, making it a weekly practice might work best. You may find that doing it in the morning while drinking a cup of coffee works well. Others may prefer doing it right before bed, as that allows them to reflect on the entire day. This time of day may also help you quiet your mind before bed. Through trial and error, you will find what works for you. Making writing a routine is more important than the time of day.

Especially when starting out, it can be beneficial to set a timer for a specific length of time, such as fifteen minutes. To help you remember, you may decide that it helps keep you on task if you set an alarm on your phone or write it in your calendar. Some people discover that having a particular ritual (or rituals) makes journaling easier to implement. For instance:

- Lighting a candle
- Dimming the lights
- Playing soft music, worship music, or a favorite song
- Drinking a cup of tea or coffee (I find that I enjoy hot chocolate, too, particularly in the winter!)
- Saying a calming prayer
- Snuggling up in a warm blanket

Whatever you choose, let it be something to help settle your mind. It's important to keep the gratitude journal someplace where you will see it, such as on your nightstand or by your favorite chair. This placement will help you remember to use it on a daily basis.

4. *Decide what to write about.* Some people will have no problem coming up with things to write about in their journals. Choosing three to five things to be grateful for each day is a good objective. However, if you have more or less on some days, that's perfectly fine, too. There are no set rules. No way is right or wrong.

Staring at a blank page can be daunting. There is no reason to overthink things. What you are thankful for can be as simple as "family," "my yummy lunch," or "the wonderful book I finished today." Try to elaborate on each one, where possible, as this can help you, over time, gain an appreciation of what's most important in your life (and what may add to your stress and be something you can cut out). Where possible, include people, too, not only objects. Instead of listing that you are grateful for your pet, elaborate. Describe something specific that you enjoy. For instance, I have a turtle. He makes me smile on a daily basis, for so many reasons. I often write about him in my journal: "I'm grateful for Speedy, who makes me smile every time I see him peeking out from under his rock to see what I'm up to."

Don't just go through the motions and hurry in order to be able to cross one more item off your to-do list. Look at this activity as developing an attitude of gratitude. Reflect for a few moments on what you are writing about.

When you're just starting out, you may find it helpful to use prompts. Here are some simple prompts to get you started on:

- Write about someone who did something nice for you.

- Write about something that makes you unique for which you're grateful.
- Write about something you're looking forward to.
- Write about the last time you laughed until you cried.
- Write about three people who've helped you through tough situations.
- Write about a time you were able to help someone else.
- Write about something that made you smile.
- Write about a loved one.
- Write about the last time you were silly.
- Write about something you see outside your window for which you're grateful.
- Write about something you can do now that you weren't able to do five years ago.
- Write about something you know now that you didn't know before your illness/pain began for which you're thankful.
- Write about your favorite childhood memory.
- Write about one thing for which you're grateful, such as a house, car, pet, job, etc.
- Write about your favorite sight, sound, and smell.

5. *Find what works for you.* With gratitude journaling, there are no set rules. You're the only person who will see your journal (unless you choose to share it with others). You can do anything you want in it to express yourself. Some people like to write, while others enjoy adding photos or drawing pictures. In fact, you could do all three!

The benefits gained from gratitude journaling are endless. You may find that by making it a regular practice, it's easier to notice that silver lining on days where you're having a flare-up. Journaling will not magically make your pain or problems disappear. But by writing regularly, your mind will learn to look for the positives throughout the course of each day, as well as tune in to the many blessings going on around you on a daily basis. It's a matter of changing your mind's channel.

Some people find it helpful to start the morning by reading over what they wrote the prior day. This could work in reverse, too. If you find that writing in the morning works best for you, then before you went to bed, you could reread what you journaled. In doing so, you are bookending your day with gratitude.

Remember what it says in Philippians 4:8-9:

> *And now, dear brothers and sisters, one final thing. Fix your thoughts on what is true, and honorable, and right, and pure, and lovely, and admirable. Think about things that are excellent and worthy of praise. Keep putting into practice all you learned and received from me—everything you heard from me and saw me doing. Then the God of peace will be with you.*

6. *Download gratitude journaling apps.* Some people love technology, and they may prefer using an app instead of a physical notebook. If this sounds like you, here are some apps you may want to check out:

- Gratitude (www.gratefulness.me): This app includes daily doses of inspiring affirmations and quotes, letters of gratitude, daily reminders, and even photo attachments. It's available for Android and iPhone.

- Live Happy (www.livehappy.com): This app is from the makers of *Live Happy* magazine. It's not just focused on gratitude journaling. It provides tips from psychologists and others to help you live a happier, healthier life. There are also shows and interviews you can watch on various topics, including gratitude, mindfulness, and overall well-being. It's available for Android and iPhone.

- 365 Gratitude (https://365gratitudejournal.com): This is not just a journaling app. It contains daily challenges, as well as daily prompts, the latter of which is designed to help you appreciate your relationships with family and friends. There is a mindfulness feature, as well as a community feature, where you can connect with and support others. A mood-tracking feature can be utilized to monitor your daily moods. It's available for Android and iPhone.

- Day One Journal (https://dayoneapp.com): This app contains a digital journal where you can store photos and videos. You can set notifications and reminders. There is a subscription plan available. There is also a component that is geared toward developing habits of gratitude and mindfulness. It's available for Android and iPhone.

- Grateful: A Gratitude Journal (www.treebetty.com): This app contains daily prompts that give you ideas of what to write about. You can also use your own. It's a basic app—nothing fancy—that's only available on iPhone.

- Reflectly (www.reflectly.app): Users are able to reflect upon their daily thoughts, as well as take note of their habits. Journaling prompts are provided. It's designed to help the user lower their stress levels, as well as learn gratitude, kindness, and empathy. It uses the psychological practices of mindfulness and CBT (cognitive behavioral therapy). There's a subscription option available. It's available for Android and iPhone.

7. *Give it time.* It can take a minimum of three weeks to establish a new habit. Give this practice of gratitude journaling at least twenty-one days of daily writing before deciding if this is an activity that works for you and is beneficial.

APPENDIX D

Deep Breathing

(Square Breathing)

Pain can increase our stress levels, and stress can increase our pain levels. Therefore, learning how to reduce stress can be beneficial in helping manage chronic pain. One such technique is commonly referred to as square breathing.

Square breathing is a practice of taking slow, deep breaths. It's designed to shift the focus to the breath, instead of focusing on the pain or stressful situation. Deep breathing can also be helpful in easing anxiety.

Before you start this practice, it's best to be in a comfortable position, such as sitting in a cozy chair with your feet on the floor. You want to be in a quiet, stress-free environment, if possible, so you can concentrate on your breathing. Place your hands in a relaxed position, perhaps folded in your lap. Be sure you are sitting up as straight as possible, as this will help maximize the deep breath.

Steps for Square Breathing

1. Sit upright with your hands and body in as comfortable a position as possible.
2. Exhale slowly through your mouth, releasing all the air in your lungs.
3. Inhale slowly and deeply through your nose. Take a deep "belly breath" (also known as breathing with your diaphragm). Do

this while mentally counting slowly to four. Focus on the air completely filling your lungs and abdominal cavity.

4. Hold your breath and slowly count to four.

5. Exhale through your mouth while silently counting to four. Focus on expelling all the air from your lungs.

6. Hold your breath for a count of four.

7. Repeat steps three through six.

8. Ideally, you will want to do this cycle for four repetitions. As you learn to listen to your body, it will become clear if a longer period of practice is needed or beneficial. (Some people may also find that it's more comfortable to do a different count than four. Use whatever feels most relaxing to you.)

9. Do this throughout the day, as needed.

Abdominal breathing is not the typical way of breathing for some people. Our on-the-go society does many things quickly, including breathing. It's common to breathe primarily in the chest, which is shallow breathing. Such breathing can lead to increased feelings of stress and anxiety. It does take practice to shift your breathing to your abdomen. But the change, and benefit, is noticeable almost immediately.

I have a sound machine and a relaxation app that I use regularly to aid with my deep breathing exercises. I also have a feature on my smartwatch that uses a growing and shrinking circle along with a relaxing tone. It allows me to sync my breath to the action.

No matter which way you choose to do this activity, take your time. Some beginners may find that they feel a bit dizzy the first time doing this. If that's the case, stop when that happens. Take things at a slower pace and gradually increase the time you spend on deep breathing. The important part is to focus on your breath, not how long you breathe in, out, or hold your breath. The more you practice, the easier it will become.

MY STORY

My health may fail, and my spirit may grow weak,
but God remains the strength of my heart; he is mine forever.

—Psalm 73:26

October 26, 1994. That day may not mean anything to you, but it's a day I will never forget. It's the day my life changed forever. It's the day I was hit by a car. It's also the day I began my long, winding journey with chronic pain and illness, though it took me ten years to get that first diagnosis.

Chronic pain and illness are difficult roads to travel. I had been sick in the past, and I'd always recovered. So, I don't think I understood the path before me when I was finally told in 2004 I had a chronic illness. As is common with chronic illnesses, symptoms build over time. Mine fit that typical pattern, with new issues cropping up here and there. It was easy for my primary care doctor to attribute the new symptoms to other short-term illnesses. It took a specialist to see the big picture. She examined my history and determined I was dealing with a much larger issue.

Over the years, I've asked God a lot of questions. *Why me? Why can't I have something with a simple cure? Why do I have to have an invisible illness? Why do I look perfectly fine on the outside, despite what I'm feeling on the inside? What about my dreams? Will they ever come to fruition?* It's been over twenty-five years. I still don't have answers to these and a host of other questions. I've questioned God—a lot—which is normal. I've shared my fears with Him. I've searched for meaning, peace, and acceptance. It didn't happen overnight, but I've realized that God has plans for me—big plans, in fact. His are just different than the plans I had growing up. Some of those childhood dreams did occur, just not in the way I'd originally envisioned. And that's not necessarily a bad thing. I have also been able to witness how He has used my experiences, including my pain, to prepare me for where I am now and what I am doing.

Lessons Learned

> *"Don't be dejected and sad, for the joy of the Lord is your strength!"*
>
> —Nehemiah 8:10

Since 1994, I have learned how much I need God in my life. I have also observed on many occasions how He is with me—every painful step along the way. In fact, I can't imagine navigating this journey without Him. I've had to accept that I need to ask for help—from God and those around me. That's been challenging, as I've always been independent. I don't like to admit when I'm unable to do something. However, now my body and mind remind me daily that there are things beyond my control. I've also learned how important it is to count my blessings, even those that seem tiny or insignificant. I've discovered that it's possible to have peace, joy, and hope, even on my bad flare-up days.

Over the years, I've gotten better at focusing on the positives. Some days are easier than others. Here are a few quotes I remind myself of on a regular basis. I have some of them written on sticky notes and placed around my house.

- Pain is temporary and doesn't have to control my life.
- Pain may be real, but so is hope.
- Pain is not fatal.
- Pain may test me, but I won't let it win.
- Pain will pass.
- God will give me what I need to handle the pain.
- God will provide all I need to thrive versus just survive.

That last point is key. In fact, this book stemmed, in part, out of that realization. I've been a Christ-follower since I was a child. Since my diagnosis, I've discovered how important it is to have the "peace, which exceeds anything we can understand" (Phil. 4:7)—the peace that only Jesus can provide. I've seen the Lord in the middle of many storms that threatened to dampen my spirits. During my twenty-five-year-plus battle with chronic pain and illness, I've spent a lot of time in the Word. I've clung to a number of verses to see me through the difficult times. These verses helped me to find and have HOPE (Hanging On to Positive Expectations) amid the pain.

Invisible Illnesses

The Lord is my strength and my song; he has given me victory.

—Exodus 15:2

My diagnoses fall under the term "invisible illness," which is an umbrella term used to describe medical conditions that aren't easily visible to others. Those illnesses may last years or even a lifetime. There is typically no cure, though the conditions may go into remission for a time. While chronic in nature, illnesses vary in severity and can present differently from person to person. With symptoms that wax and wane daily, or even hourly, making plans can be challenging. Some people are able to live an active, somewhat "normal" life, while others are largely homebound. Symptoms or medication side effects may make it next to impossible to get out of bed or perform basic daily tasks.

Chronic illness includes physical conditions, such as arthritis, fibromyalgia, asthma, adrenal fatigue, migraines, diabetes, Crohn's, cancer, high blood pressure, Lyme disease, chronic obstructive pulmonary disease (COPD), multiple sclerosis (MS), lupus, chronic fatigue syndrome (CFS), epilepsy, POTS (Postural Orthostatic Tachycardia Syndrome), IST (Inappropriate Sinus

Tachycardia), and so many more. Also included are mental illnesses, such as bipolar disorder, depression, schizophrenia, and anxiety. These illnesses are ongoing, hence the term "chronic." They could last a lifetime. But there will be ups and downs. For some, there may be predictability with symptoms and triggers. Those triggers can include weather changes, certain foods, or even stress. My biggest triggers are weather changes, heat, and stress.

Pain and fatigue often fight for my attention, particularly on days when I'm sick or hurting—and they often win. Chronic pain forces me to take inventory and focus on what's most important. Coping with the peaks and valleys is one of the hardest parts to deal with and for others to understand. However, the Lord understands (Isa. 40:28-31). He has given me strength on more than one occasion to get through the next moment. That fact alone is enough to give me—or anyone else—hope and peace.

A New Way of Life

"But forget all that—it is nothing compared to what I am going to do.
For I am about to do something new. See, I have already begun! Do you not see it?"

—Isaiah 43:18-19

For people battling a chronic illness, it's not uncommon to experience the stages of grief: denial, anger, bargaining, depression, and acceptance. And I've gone through each of these. I've grieved the life I used to have, the one I must now bear, and the dreams I fear may never come true. Loneliness, sorrow, grief, fatigue, anger, and feelings of failure and self-judgment are emotions I experience on a regular basis. As a result, it's easy for fear and doubt to take up residence in my heart and mind. On occasion, I find I am angry at myself for poor health, depressed because of the new limits on my life, and in general, sick and tired of feeling sick and tired. Sadly, I've encountered judgment and criticism from others because I look fine on the outside, so I *must* be fine on the inside or making things up. No one wants to be told it's all in their head or that they shouldn't worry about the pain and other changes in their body. Sadly, some of these comments could come from those in the medical community. I've had providers give me the runaround and dismiss my illness because there's no cure. I've been told it's something I'll have to "learn to live with." That's easy for them to say, but it's not so easy to figure out how to do it. It's particularly challenging when I suddenly feel like a character in a book with a story line I never would have chosen. However, I'm discovering it's possible to rewrite the plot.

There is often a stigma attached to chronic illness and chronic pain. I know I'm experiencing something that doesn't go away. Things feel out of control with my body. It's hard to explain things to others—including friends, family members, employers, and coworkers—when I don't even fully understand what's going on. I truly believe some of them perceived me as lazy, which couldn't be further from the truth. Others have told me that if I just "lighten up" or "exercise more," then I'll feel better. What makes the situation worse is that my symptoms ebb and flow, so that can result in challenges and delays when trying to obtain a proper diagnosis.

Over the years, pain robbed me of the smallest pleasures in life. Chronic pain causes me to feel helpless and hopeless at the loss of control I now have over so many parts of my life. In fact, the pain I'm experiencing isn't just an inconvenience. It affects my entire self, physically and mentally. My ability to do something one day may not carry over to the next. Or I could go days or weeks without a flare-up; then suddenly, I'm barely able to function. On occasion, it feels as though I'm living two separate lives. I question, at times, if the pain or illness is solely there to steal my joy, hopes, dreams, and possibly my life.

I realize it's natural to struggle with questions such as "Am I enough?" "Will I ever be who I used to be?" and "What did I do wrong?" And at times, it seems like I'm fighting a losing battle—within my body as well as with those around me.

God knows the questions on your heart. It's important to remember that you are not your illness. Hope and despair are opposite emotions, and it's natural to struggle between them. However, it *is* possible to find peace in the middle of any storm if you have the Lord on your side. Your hope is in Him. It does not depend on your physical or mental health. With Him, you can survive *and* thrive.

Keys for My Hope

You are the light of the world—like a city on a hilltop that cannot be hidden. No one lights a lamp and then puts it under a basket. Instead, a lamp is placed on a stand, where it gives light to everyone in the house.

—Matthew 5:14-15

Here are some keys I use to help me hold on to hope while living with chronic pain and illness:

- I acknowledge that the nature of my illness changes. It's rarely predictable. However, I can always depend on the Lord to be there. That *never* changes.
- I spend quiet time with the Lord. I take time to pray and listen to what He wants to say to me, as well as read His Word. I've found a routine that works and allows me to remain consistent with this practice.
- I focus on the good, too. I still have a lot to offer. I can help others by sharing my story, offering coping tips, etc. I am confident God will use my situation for His good as I reflect His presence in my life.
- I try not to isolate myself. Family and friends want to help and be there for me, if only to listen. I've learned to allow them to do so.

- Finally, I remember that I am a survivor. Through my battle with chronic pain and illness, I've faced many trials. But I've also found strength, insight, and resilience that others may not experience.

Living with chronic pain and illness is not easy. Thankfully, I never have to go through it alone. And neither do you.

RESOURCES

American Cancer Society: www.cancer.org

American Chronic Pain Association: www.theacpa.org

American Diabetes Association: www.diabetes.org

American Heart Association: www.heart.org

American Lung Association: www.lung.org

American Migraine Foundation: www.americanmigrainefoundation.org

Anxiety and Depression Association of America: www.adaa.org

Arthritis Foundation: www.arthritis.org

Asthma and Allergy Foundation of America: www.aafa.org

Chronic Disease Coalition: www.chronicdiseasecoalition.org

COPD Foundation: www.copdfoundation.org

Crohn's and Colitis Foundation: www.crohnscolitisfoundation.org

Depression and Bipolar Support Alliance: www.dbsalliance.org

Dysautonomia International: www.dysautonomiainternational.org

Epilepsy Foundation: www.epilepsy.com

IACFS/ME (International Association of Chronic Fatigue Syndrome/ Myalgic Encephalomyelitis): www.iacfsme.org

International Bipolar Foundation: www.ibpf.org

Invisible Disabilities Association: www.invisibledisabilities.org

Lupus Foundation of America: www.lupus.org

Lyme Disease Association: www.lymediseaseassociation.org

National Association on Mental Illness: www.nami.org

National Fibromyalgia and Chronic Pain Association: www.ibroandpain.org

National Headache Foundation: www.headaches.org

National Multiple Sclerosis Society: www.nationalmssociety.org

Schizophrenia and Related Disorders Alliance of America: www.sardaa.org

The Mighty: www.themighty.com

US Pain Foundation: www.uspainfoundation.org

SCRIPTURE VERSES

This is a list of the verses used in this book. They have encouraged me along my journey, and I hope they can encourage you, as well.

Old Testament

Genesis 1:27

Genesis 2:3

Exodus 15:2

Deuteronomy 3:18

Joshua 1:9

1 Samuel 17:37

1 Chronicles 16:11

2 Chronicles 1:3-4

2 Chronicles 4:17

2 Chronicles 9:8

2 Chronicles 12:9

2 Chronicles 15:7

Nehemiah 8:10

Job 42:2

Psalm 2:13

Psalm 4:1

Psalm 4:13

Psalm 13:5

Psalm 18:16–19

Psalm 25:1–2

Psalm 25:16

Psalm 27:14

Psalm 46:10

Psalm 56:3

Psalm 61:2–3

Psalm 62:5

Psalm 63:6-8

Psalm 73:26

Psalm 105:4

Psalm 138:8

Psalm 139:2–3

Psalm 139:5

Psalm 139:13–14

Proverbs 16:24

Isaiah 26:3

Isaiah 33:6

Isaiah 40:29

Isaiah 41:10

Isaiah 43:1

Isaiah 43:18–19

Isaiah 62:3

Daniel 3:17

Habakkuk 3:18

Habakkuk 3:19

New Testament

Matthew 5:14-15

Matthew 6:34

Matthew 11:28

Mark 4:39

Mark 5:3-4

Mark 11:24

Luke 5:16

Luke 6:38

Luke 12:6-7

Luke 12:30-31

Luke 22:42

John 11:35

John 14:27

John 16:32

Acts 3:20

Romans 5:5

Romans:5:8

Romans 8:18

Romans 8:28

Romans 8:31

Romans 9:20

Romans 12:12

2 Corinthians 1:3

2 Corinthians 5:17

Ephesians 3:16

Philippians 1:6

Philippians 3:8–9

Philippians 4:7

Philippians 4:8

Philippians 4:9

Philippians 4:11–12

Philippians 4:13

Philippians 18:39

1 Thessalonians 5:16–18

2 Timothy 1:7

2 Timothy 4:7

Hebrews 13:8

James 1:2–4

James 3:2

James 3:7–8

1 Peter 5:7

1 John 3:1

1 John 5:14–15

ACKNOWLEDGMENTS

Writing this book was something I never could've imagined a few years ago. I've always felt uncomfortable sharing my story. Yet God had other plans. I hesitated to include this page for fear I'd leave someone out. Sadly, I probably did. But I want you to know that if you have crossed my path at some point in time, I know it was for a reason, and I thank you.

First and foremost, I want to thank the Lord for giving me the words to say. Thank You for using my weaknesses for Your glory. When the pain overwhelms me, thank You for understanding the cries of my heart and never leaving my side. Thank You for being my hope and giving me the strength to get through each moment of every day.

To my husband, Jeff, you have been with me throughout this entire journey and all the ups and downs. You are my best friend, the love of my life, my helper, and my biggest supporter. Thank you for loving me unconditionally. You believe in me, and you have encouraged me to keep going when I've wanted to give up. God surely knew what He was doing when He sent you across my path at Behrend. You are a true gift from God.

To my family, thank you for your love, encouragement, and prayers over the years.

To Poppa, who has been with the Lord since 1996. Though you're not here physically to see this book, I have no doubt you're watching over me, as you have my entire life. You are deeply loved and missed.

To my editor, Katie Cruice Smith, thank you for helping me fine-tune my message.

To Ambassador International, thank you for believing in my words/ vision/book and for giving me the opportunity to fulfill a lifelong dream of being a published author. It's been such a joy to work with all of you.

To Dori Harrell, thank you for your edits and guidance.

To Christina Lorenzen, thanks for your support and encouragement. You made 2020 a bit more bearable! Words can't express how much I value our friendship.

To the ladies in the Hope Amid the Pain Facebook group and the online chronic pain community, thank you for your support. It's such a blessing to connect with others who are familiar with the challenges associated with chronic pain and illness and are able to remind each other that we're not alone. The Lord is with us!

To my early endorsers: Debbie Macomber, Rachel Van Dyken, Patricia J. Edwards, Amy Clipston, Elizabeth Byler Younts, Amanda Barratt, Heidi Chiavaroli, Susan Sleeman, Kathleen Fuller, Sharee Stover, Candace Calvert, and Vannetta Chapman. You encouraged me early on by helping me realize others could benefit from my story and that I didn't need to be afraid to share it.

To The King's Pen writers' group, thank you for your friendship and encouragement to share my story, knowing that God had plans to use it all for His glory.

And finally, to my readers, thank you for following me on this journey. I pray you find comfort and hope in God's Word as You draw closer to Him.

For more information about

Leslie L. McKee
and
Hope Amid the Pain
please visit:

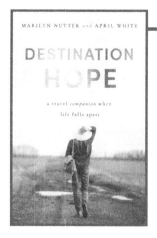

MARILYN NUTTER and APRIL WHITE

DESTINATION HOPE

a travel companion when
life falls apart

Destination Hope is a must-read invaluable guide, offering hope and sound wisdom for your unpredictable, individual life journeys. Written by two of the wisest tried, tested, and true women of God—April White and Marilyn Nutter—you will see how each author poured out beautiful transparency. Like two best friends who've trailed the hard ground before you, April and Marilyn, seem to gently take you by the hand and lead you toward God's heart for healing.

In *Chronic Love*, Brooke Bartz reveals a deeply raw and descriptive account of life with a chronic and debilitating illness, and she shares with readers how comfort and strength can be found through the Truth in God's Word. Specifically designed for women who daily battle chronic illness, Chronic Love's goal is to provide solid Scriptural encouragement for the fight.

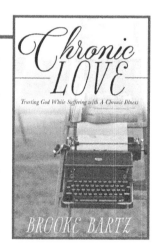

Chronic LOVE

Trusting God While Suffering with A Chronic Illness

BROOKE BARTZ

YET
WILL
I
PRAISE
HIM

LIVING AND PARENTING WITH A CHRONIC ILLNESS

Hannah Wingert

After finally being diagnosed with a chronic illness following the birth of her fourth child, Hannah has had to come to terms with her diagnosis and to learn to be a wife and mother in the midst of her invisible illness. In her inspirational book, *Yet Will I Praise Him,* Hannah opens up candidly about her own struggles of living and parenting with a chronic illness.

Made in the USA
Las Vegas, NV
31 October 2021

33413531R00098